Stoplights Are For Laughing

Easy Ways to Keep Laughter in Your Life

BONNIE B. DANEKER

Illustrated by Eevie Lanier

Stoplights Are For Laughing: Easy Ways to Keep Laughter in Your Life

Bonnie B. Daneker, author

ISBN: 978-0-9910032-5-9 (Paperback)

ISBN: 978-0-9910032-7-3 (eBook)

Illustrations by Eevie Lanier

Book design by Becky's Graphic Design®, LLC
www.BeckysGraphicDesign.com

Printed in U.S.A

To my girlfriends and guyfrends,
who bring joy through laughter and love

How this book began

I grew up in a small—but growing—town in Northeastern Ohio. In our neighborhood, the kids would often gather for games like Wiffleball, Kick-the-Can, Tag, and Kickball. On a corner lot, our home was the "Kool-Aid House" where we would play and laugh, being rewarded for staying out of our parents' hair with an icy pitcher of punch (and sometimes cookies). We had a lot of fun.

We kids also saw many of our parents socialize, travel, and work together. Another of my favorite memories is an event put on by my parents' social group. Called the "Laugh Olympics," it featured somewhat ridiculous games they created (like pushing a cucumber with your nose across the finish line) which led to more laughter than progress.

Now that I am an adult, I see friendships and laughter as two critical components to a fulfilled life. I'm thrilled that I still have friends from those childhood days. Now, my friends live in different cities and time zones, with different lives. We know we don't have to talk every day or demonstrate our ability to move vegetables, but we could if we wanted to. And that's the beauty of loving friendships: If you nurture them a little, you can just pick up where you left off, no matter how much time has passed!

This book is written to give you some ideas to sustain love in those friendships, based on experiences I have had or known about. When we have the chance to celebrate our friendships, we should do so!

With Love, Bonnie B. Daneker

P.S. By all means, make these ideas your own! Send in other suggestions or comments to me on the *Stoplights Book Series* Facebook page.

Stoplights
Are For Laughing

1
Laugh at the stoplights

This collection of engaging ideas is named for a very simple one: Laughing together in the car, especially at stop signs or stoplights. With all of the other To-Dos in your life, taking the time to be with your bestie is among the most valuable—and laughing together is priceless. When you're riding in the car, it sometimes doesn't matter where you're driving to: You could be road-tripping or carpooling to work, but you're enjoying being together, making jokes, competing in drive-time trivia, or playing "remember when." Laughing makes the time go faster and it's a lot more fun!

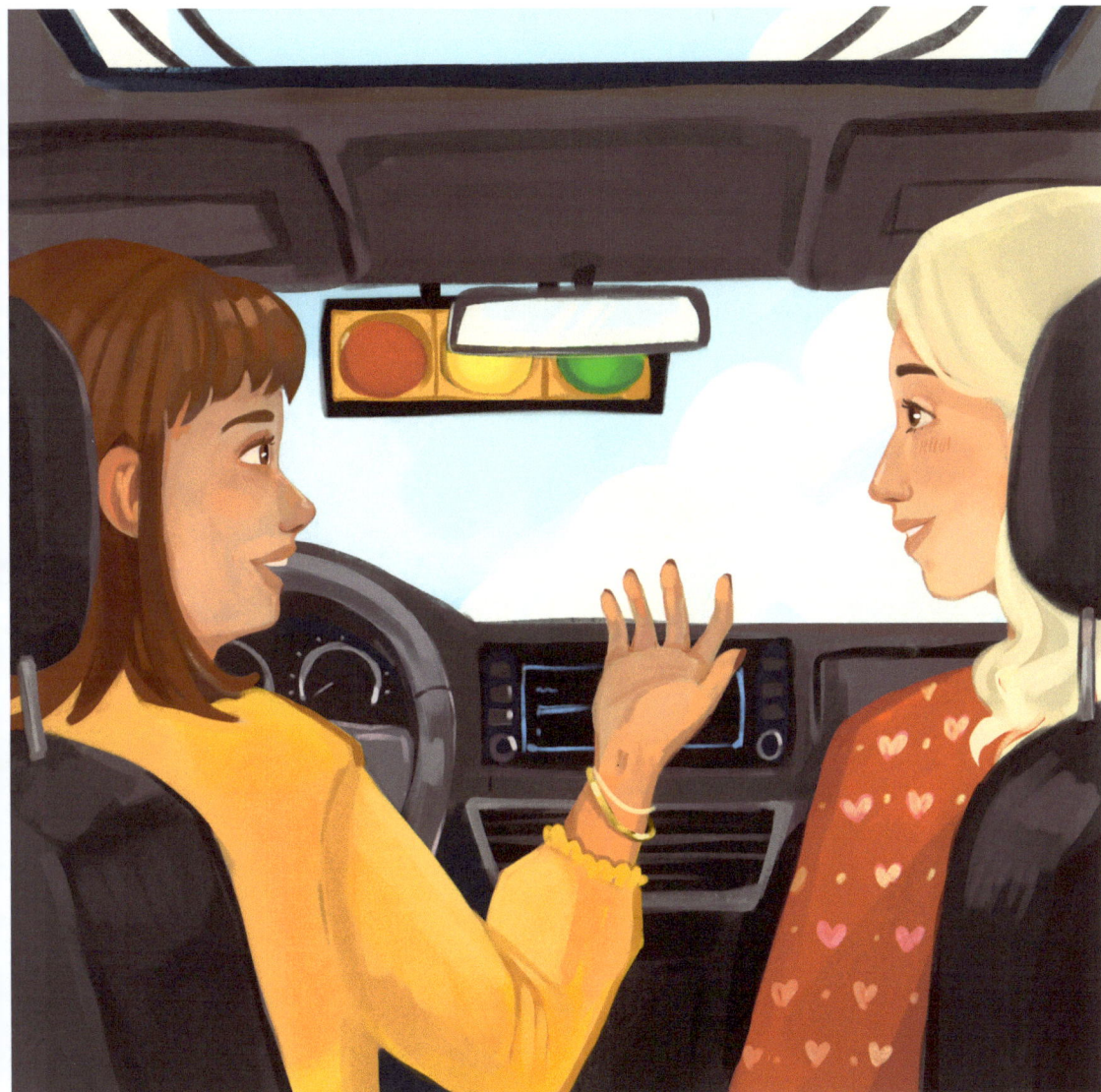

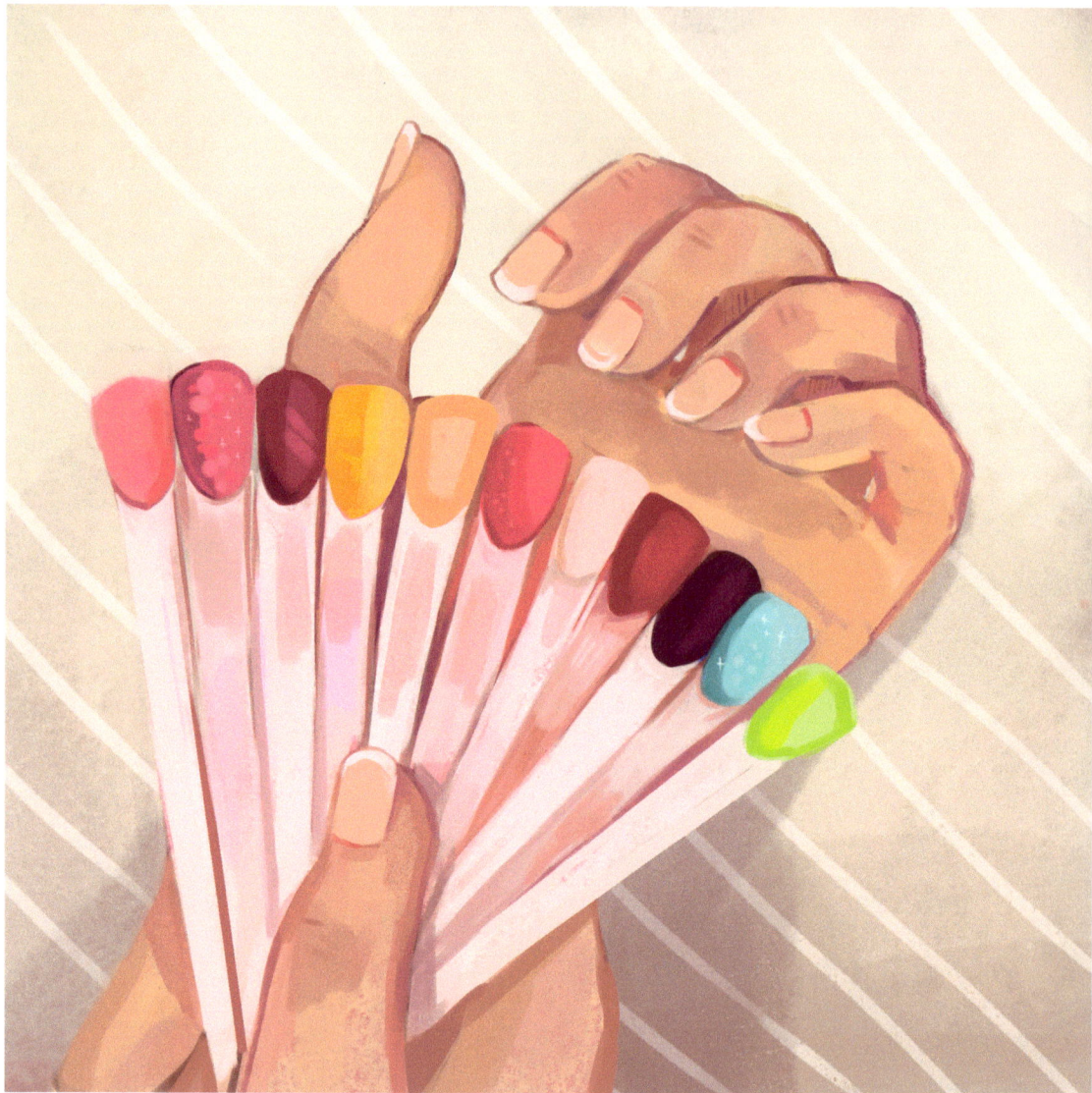

2
Choose colors for a mani-pedi

One of my girlfriends is fastidious about nail care. She maintains a weekly appointment at her favorite salon and requests precise nail shapes. One thing she does change up is her colors. If my schedule coincides with hers, I make it a point to meet up. Picking colors and treatments is made even more likeable when you're doing it with a friend. We consider holidays (copper or burgundy for Thanksgiving?) and seasons (summer white or yellow?) as well as finishes (chrome, glitter, or ombre?). Sometimes I'll pick hers or she'll pick mine, and the results can get crazy, but what are friends for?

3

Buy bath salts to share and compare

Hydrotherapy has been around for thousands of years, and it's no wonder: it works. Most appreciate the therapeutic goodness of warm water, which is often made even more magical with wonderfully-scented salts, bombs and bubble baths. During the pandemic when we couldn't go shopping together in person, one of my friends and I would compare bath products online. She would buy one, and I another, reporting on which we liked. We'd evaluate their moisturizing or cleansing ingredients, fragrance, and availability. When we both liked them, if they were packaged in quantity (like an eight-pack), we would sometimes split half the package.

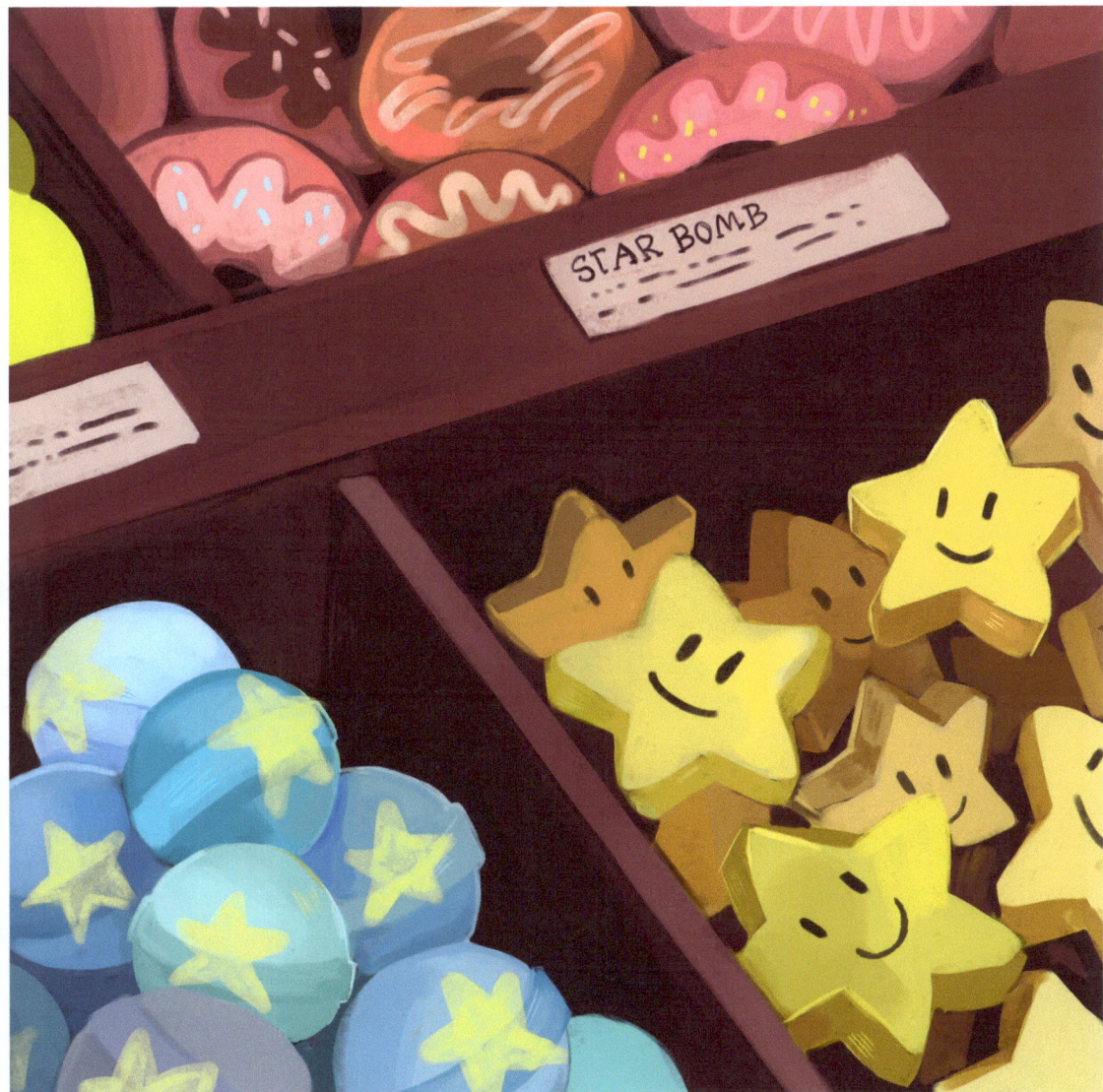

STAR BOMB

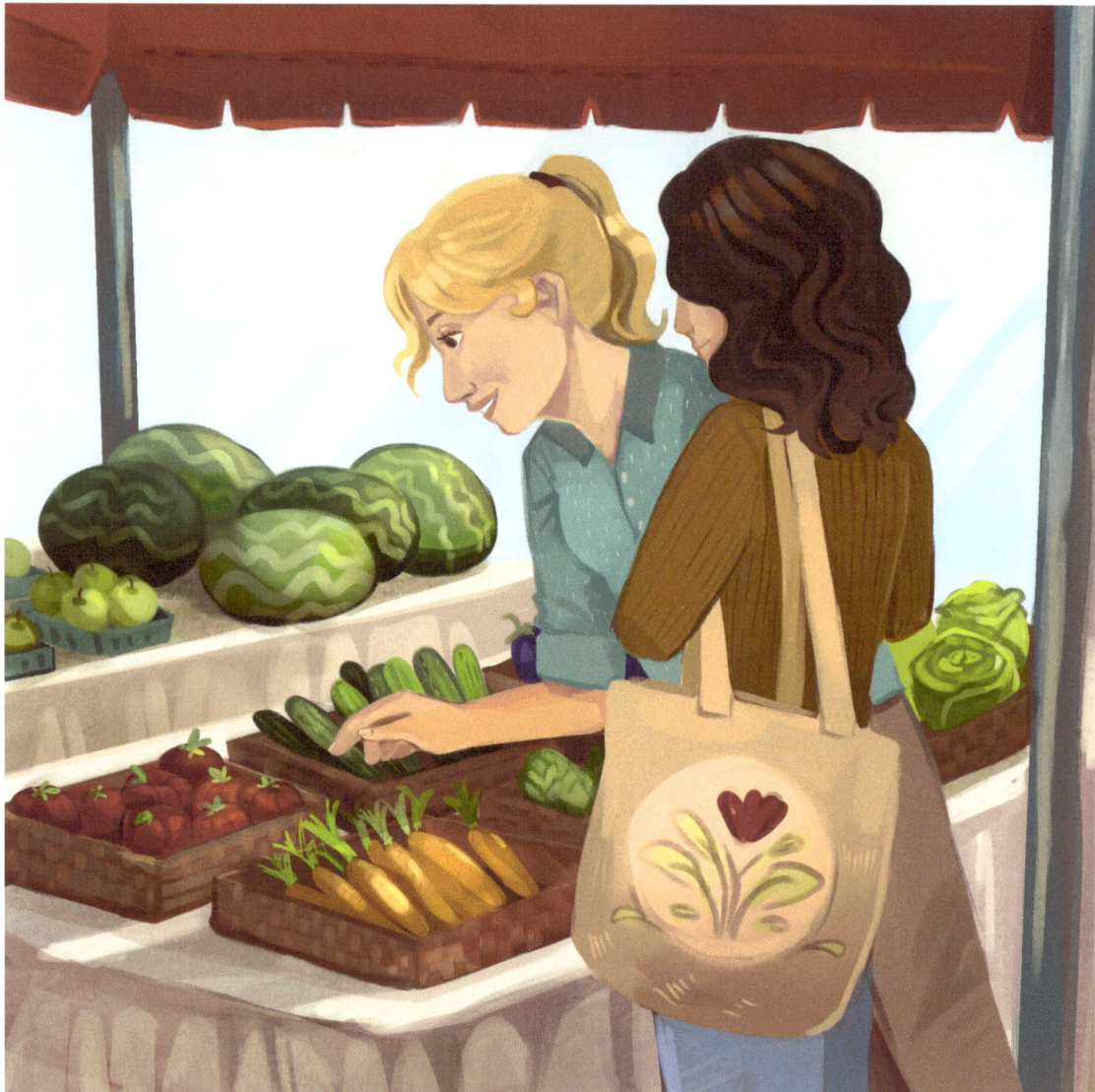

4
Frequent farmer's markets

My love of fresh fruits and vegetables is well-known among many of my friends. On early Saturday mornings between March and October, I like to go hunting for the sun-ripened agricultural goodness at local farmer's markets. Picking up a friend (especially one with a big shopping basket!) to share the experience and the bounty is a simple joy of which I never tire. Smelling perfectly-ripe heirloom tomatoes or freshly-cut herbs immediately puts me in mind of a Caprese salad with mozzarella cheese for lunch—and that's a great way to cap off the morning's shopping trip.

5

Attend a women's exhibit or female-focused film

Some of my guyfriends and family members love to see movies and shows about wars or mystical worlds. Some of my girlfriends and family members love to see those that celebrate female-centric accomplishments or stories. We all have our favorites. Most people I know, though, can agree on seeing a film or exhibit in an interesting location, like a historic movie house or pop-up space. The next time you're up for seeing a good female-focused show, find a gal pal (or guyfriend) who will enjoy attending and discussing it after with a post-show beverage.

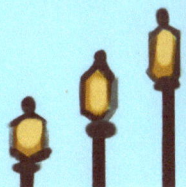

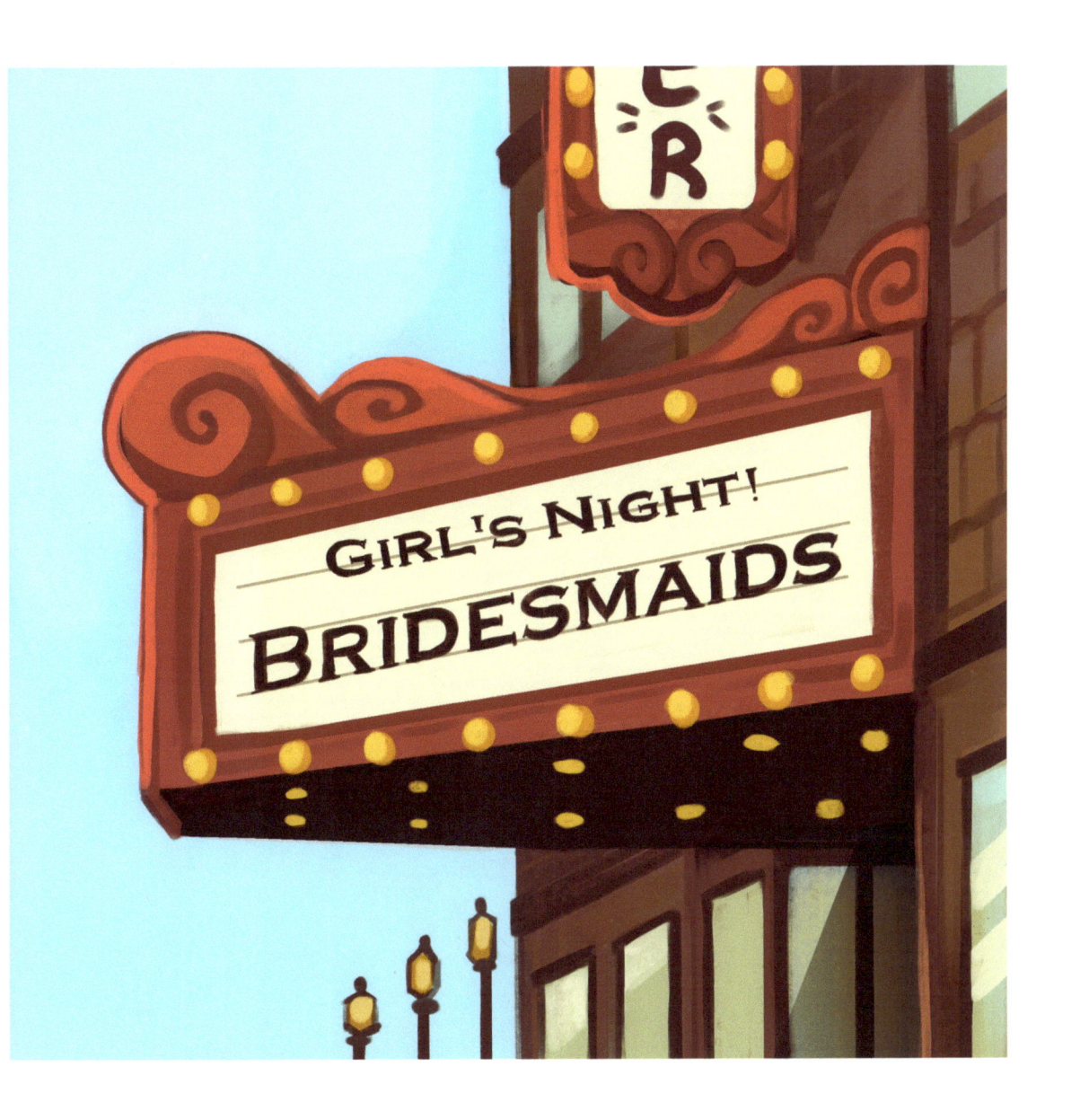

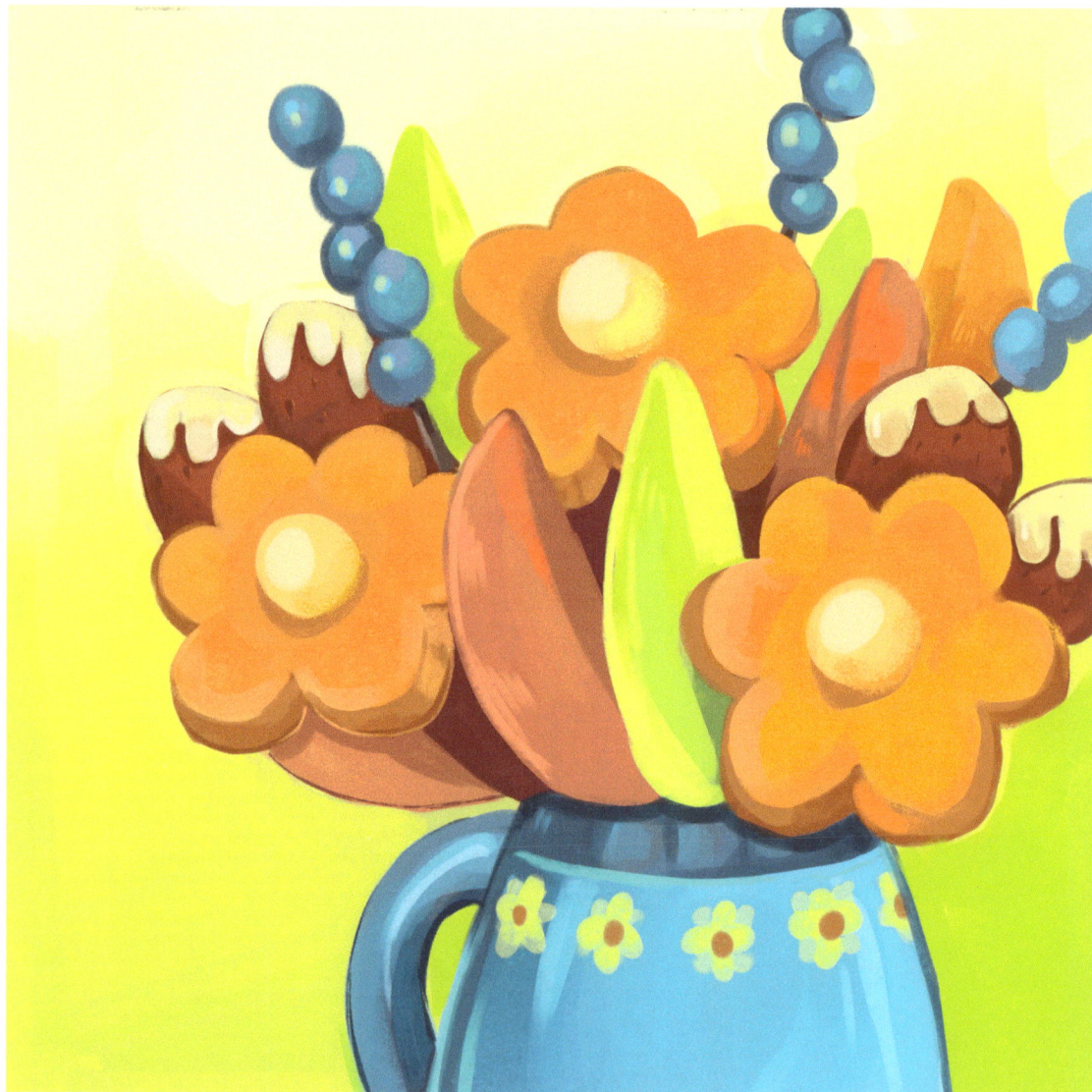

6

Deliver edible treats

Every time I see a cookie delivery van or fruit arrangement, I remember sending a very pregnant girlfriend a box of huge, gooey, chocolate chip cookies with a pint of vanilla ice cream. She called me saying she was craving that. She was due any day and too big to go out on her own, and I had it delivered to her. She and the baby were satisfied, and to this day her son loves chocolate chip cookies! If you have the chance to mark an important event or lift someone's spirits, consider sending edible treats.

7

Text news of something they care about

Have you ever gotten a text that says, "I just saw this (with a link) and thought of you!" Those texts say, "I was listening to you. I know this is important in your life. I care about you enough to make the effort to tell you so." In my mind, that's the definition of friendship. Friends may not be able to be physically nearby, but staying emotionally or mentally close is important. Keeping a connection can be simple with a quick text, and I am thankful for several friends who are terrific at that. Try it, adding emojis or .gifs too!

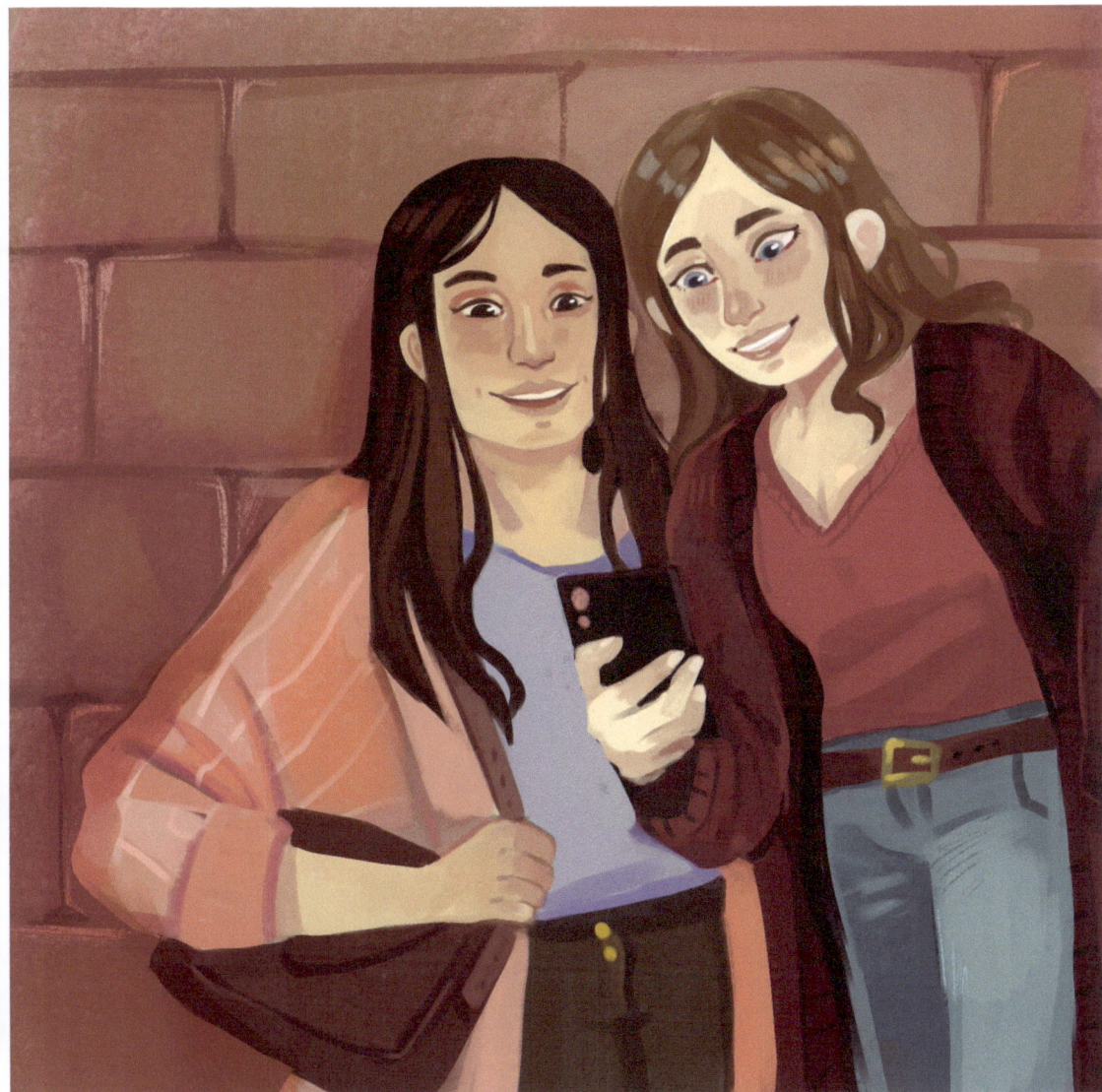

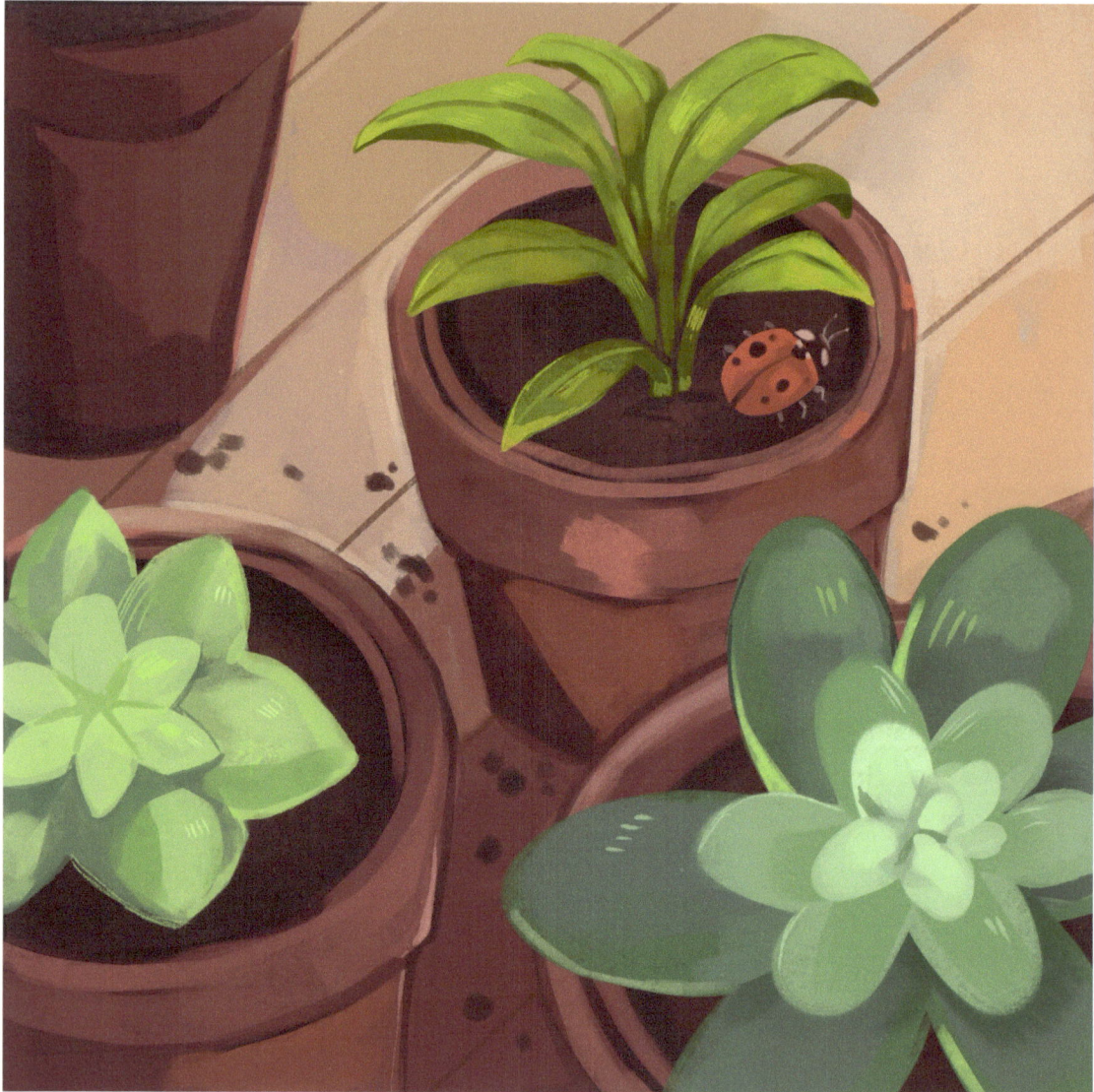

8

Give clips from your garden or indoor plants

Growing up, I was fascinated with the variety of plants my mom had on her bow window: spider plants, jade trees, violets, Swedish ivy, and Christmas cacti to name a few. They were unusual, even exotic, for our small town. I remember that she didn't usually buy these; she often received gifts of clips of plants from others. She loved both getting new ones (especially violets) and sharing the plants she had, like gifting a potted "baby spider" offshoot or some Swedish ivy growing new roots in a glass of water. So easy, and so much fun. Plus, it always gave them something to talk about!

9

Keep secrets

A true friend is one you can count on to keep your secret—
however juicy—safe. Everyone needs a person like this in
their lives: You're dying to tell someone but in today's extra
social world, most people can't be trusted, except your
A+ Secret Keeper friend. Though tempted, that friend
realizes how important it is to not tell what is going on
or how you really feel. That friend knows the importance
of shared trust, and understands that you'll be really hurt
if the secret gets out. If you are trusted with someone's
confidence, hold those secrets close to your heart.

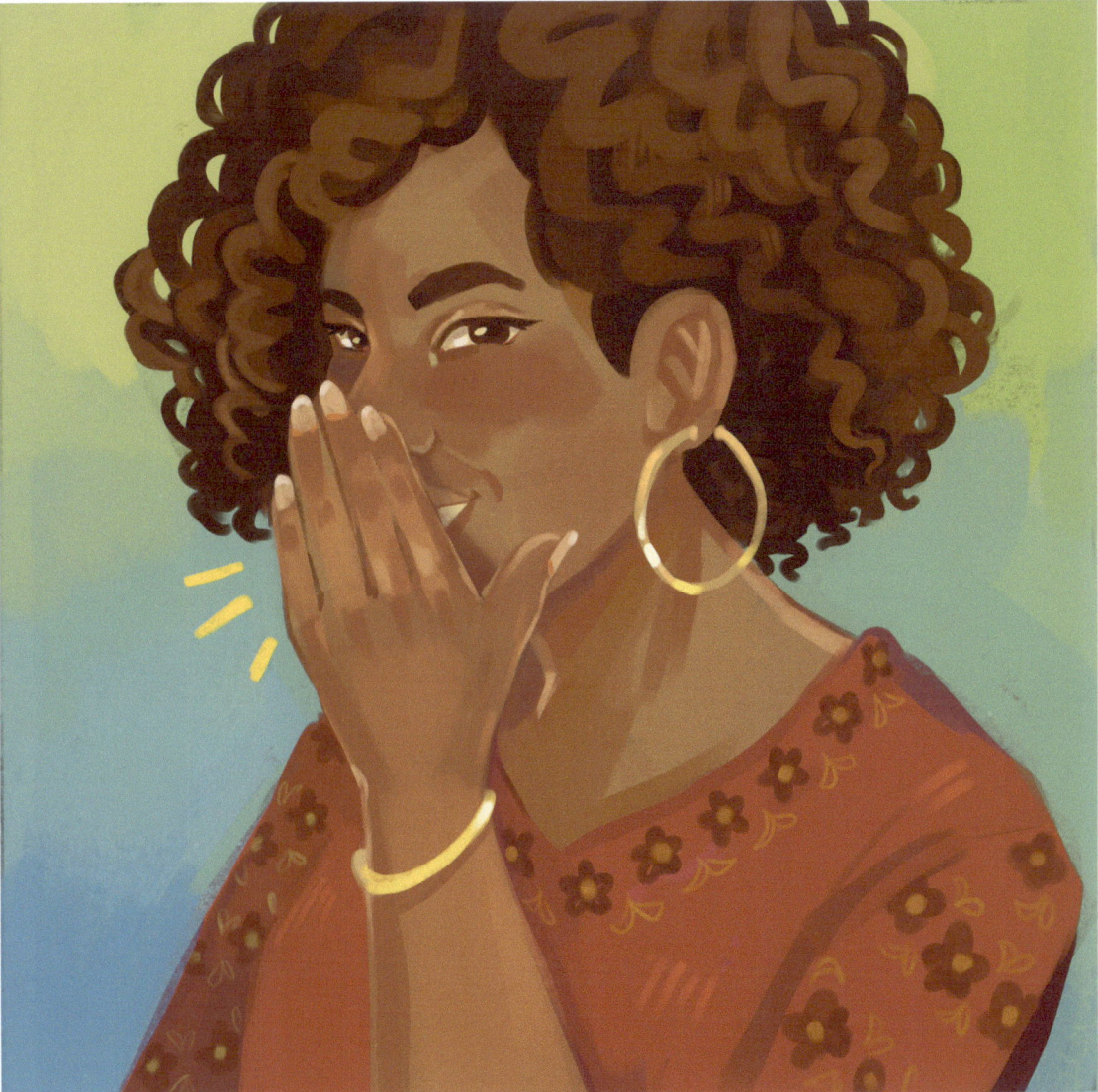

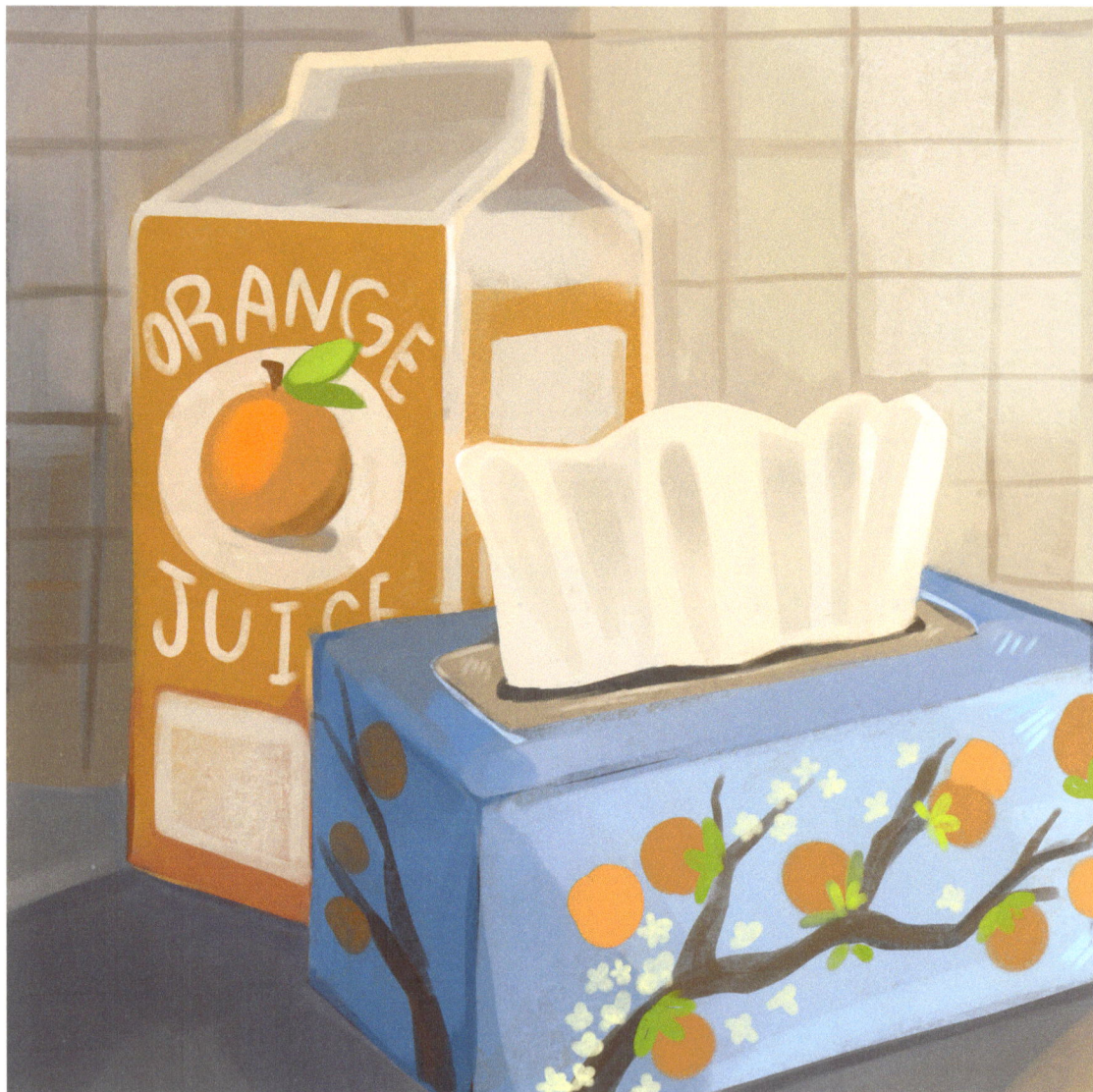

10

Bring O.J. and tissues

When you're sick with the flu, a cold, or whatever crud is going around, it's easy to feel quarantined. No one wants to catch what you have, and that's understandable. If you're ailing, you may not have the energy to launch yourself up to get to the drugstore. You may just want to stay in bed. When you call a friend to go instead and she says "No problem. What do you need?", you could start feeling better immediately. If there's a risk she could catch it herself when bringing you care goodies, she could leave them outside your door. That's what friends do.

11
Make vision boards

As a New Year's tradition, one of my friends threw a Vision Board Party: a morning beverage with girlfriends, cutting out shapes, letters, and pictures from magazines, then pasting them on a big board. The end product looked like something we would do in grade school. What made it adult-like, and more serious, is that the shapes, letters and pictures reflected our goals for the next year. The vulnerability of showing, and discussing, our vision for our futures connected us in deeper ways than I ever expected—with a bonus of suggestions and support from the others to attain those goals. What's not to like?

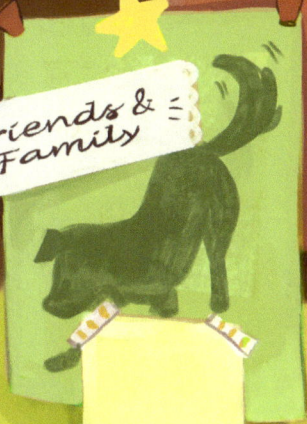

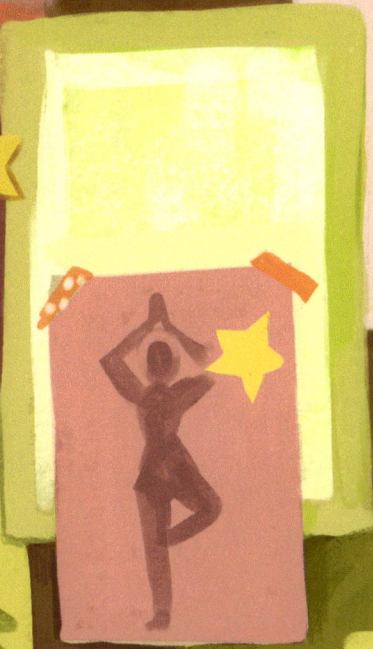

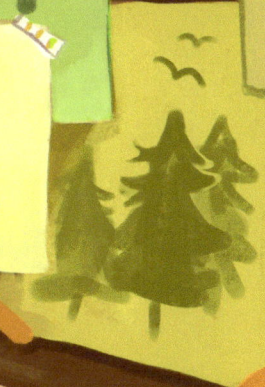

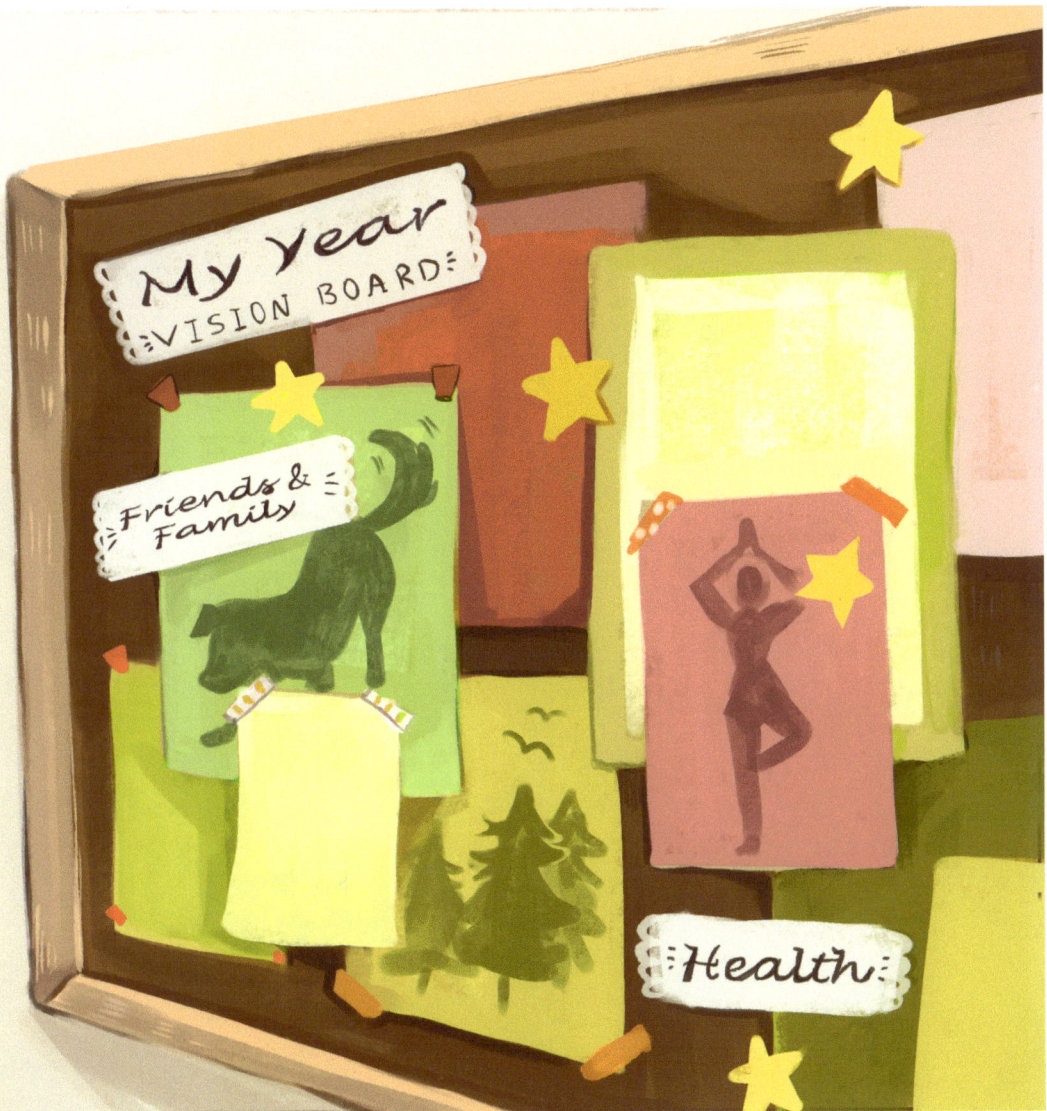

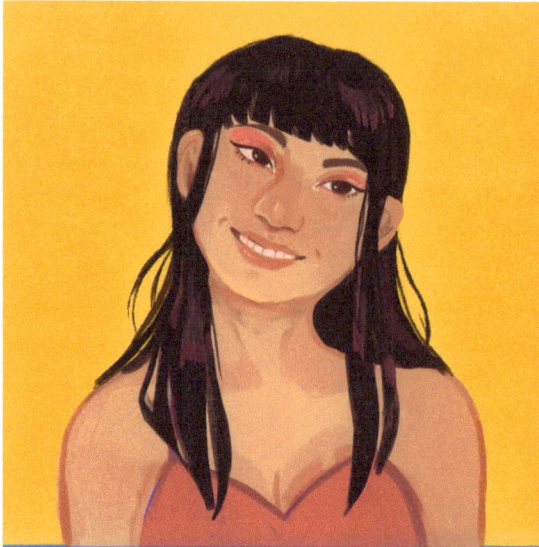

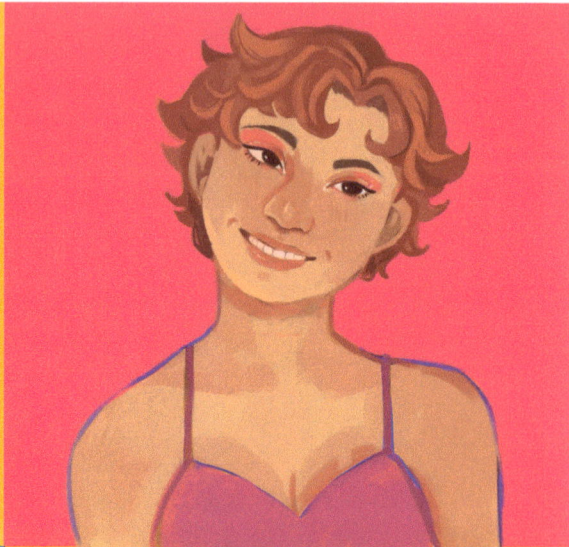

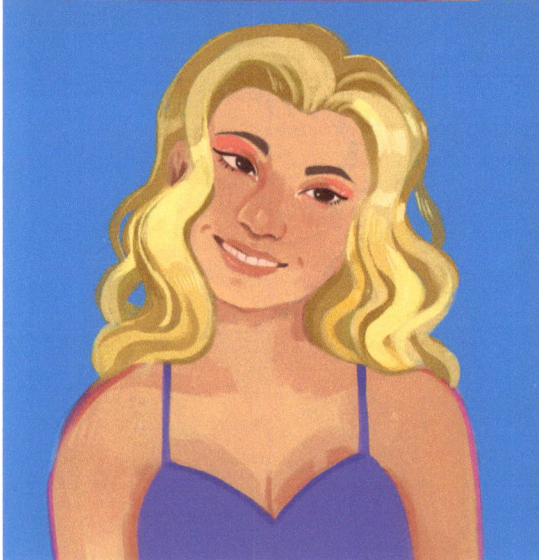

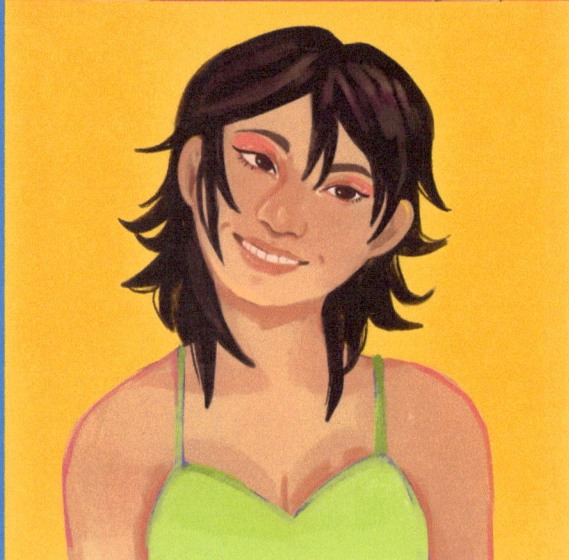

12

Shop hairstyles

As much as we may have liked the flat-ironed hair of the 2010s or the loose waves of the 2020s, we realize times change and our hairstyles do, too. Changing can be scary; after all, we have to figure out what style, what equipment, and which products to use. A talented hair professional can make the new look a reality, but it helps to go in to the salon with some ideas. Shopping online for a new 'do with a stylish friend (who you know will be brutally honest) can be unexpectedly fun—especially with the easy digital tools to show your face in a number of different styles.

13

Complete a DIY or fix-it project

Most of us are born with two arms and hands, but sometimes we just need another one (or two!). My father ambitiously bought bicycles—which needed assembly—for us kids. I helped to run brake cable, place chains on gears, and insert tire inner tubes on the 10-speeds we built. That was a great learning time for me, with the biggest lesson being, "don't tackle big projects alone." When it was time to put together my bird houses, I asked a nature-loving friend to help me out. Turns out, she was also an ace with the cordless drill and we were done in no time.

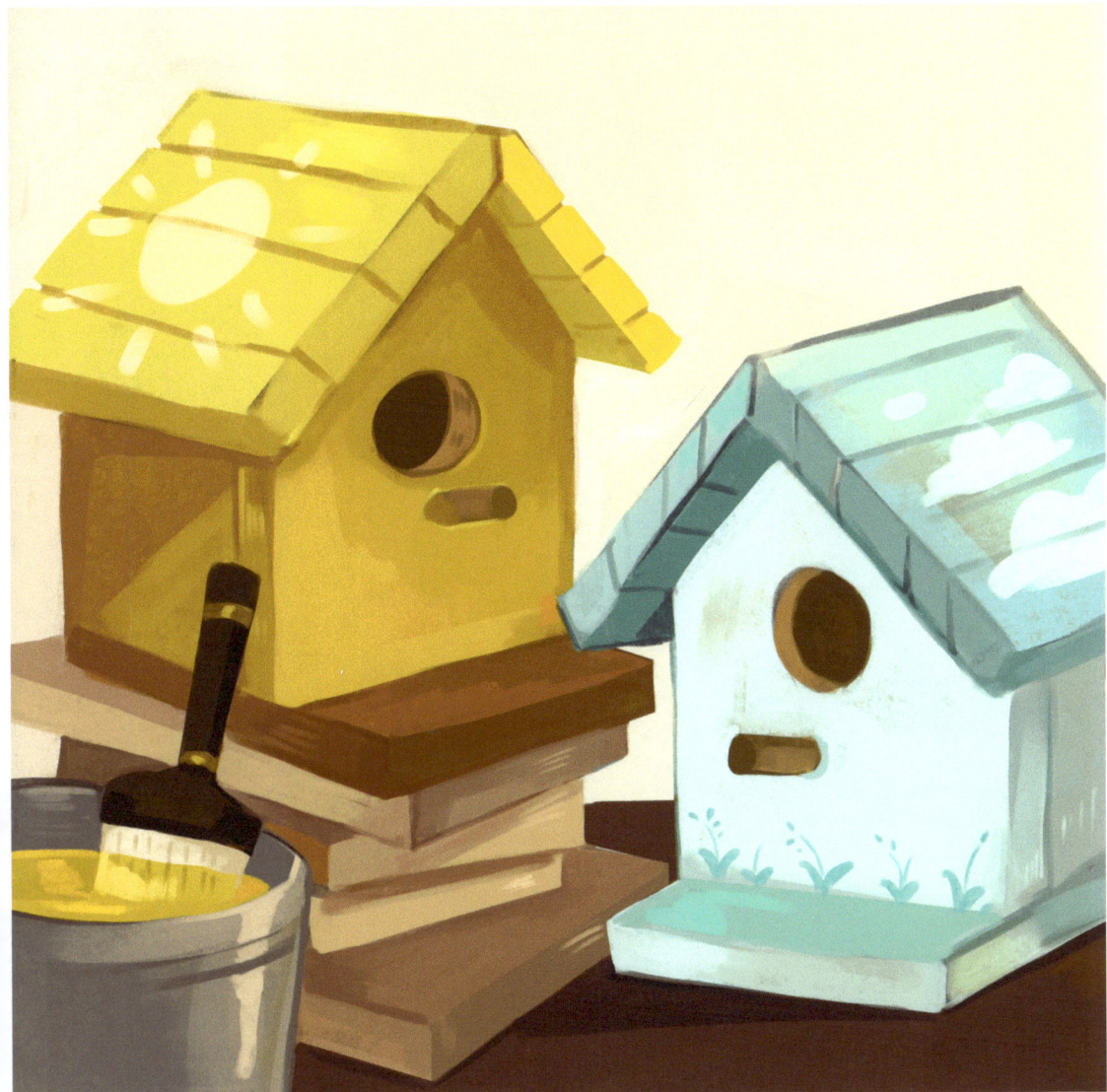

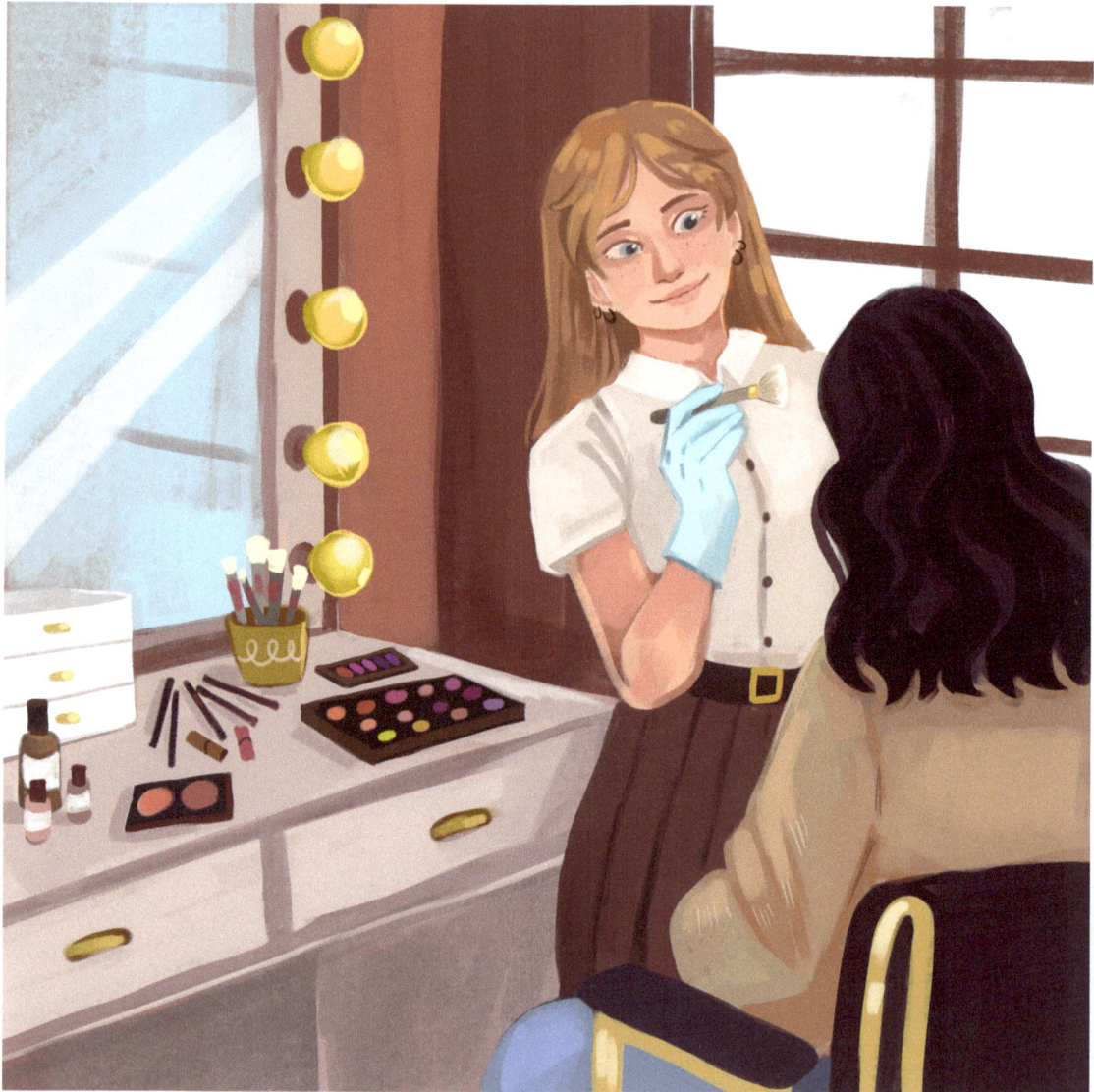

14

Get makeovers

Have you ever gone into a department store cosmetics department or makeup store and stared longingly at the shiny products? Have you ever wanted to experiment with the different brushes or colors or goop, wondering if they would work for you? Several places staff professionals whose job it is to make you look "casually-great," "evening glamorous," or "office ready" with a makeover appointment. They offer advice on what to use and how to use it. While you can go for your appointment alone, why not have an adventure with a friend?

You can both get instruction on the classics or the latest products and encourage each other to try something new.

15

Bake

Speed and convenience makes boxed meals popular, but it makes me long for the days I baked on a regular basis. You can't just throw together ingredients and have a beautiful cake, casserole, or soufflé. The chemistry and preparation are more complex than panfrying. Though it is rare, I love to invite a friend over (or head to their house) with ingredients ready to sift, measure, and stir up a new recipe. "Pre-make then bake," is a joy too, as we sometimes bring over holiday cookie dough to cut, cook, and decorate at a friend's house. Conversation is lively and cleanup is faster!

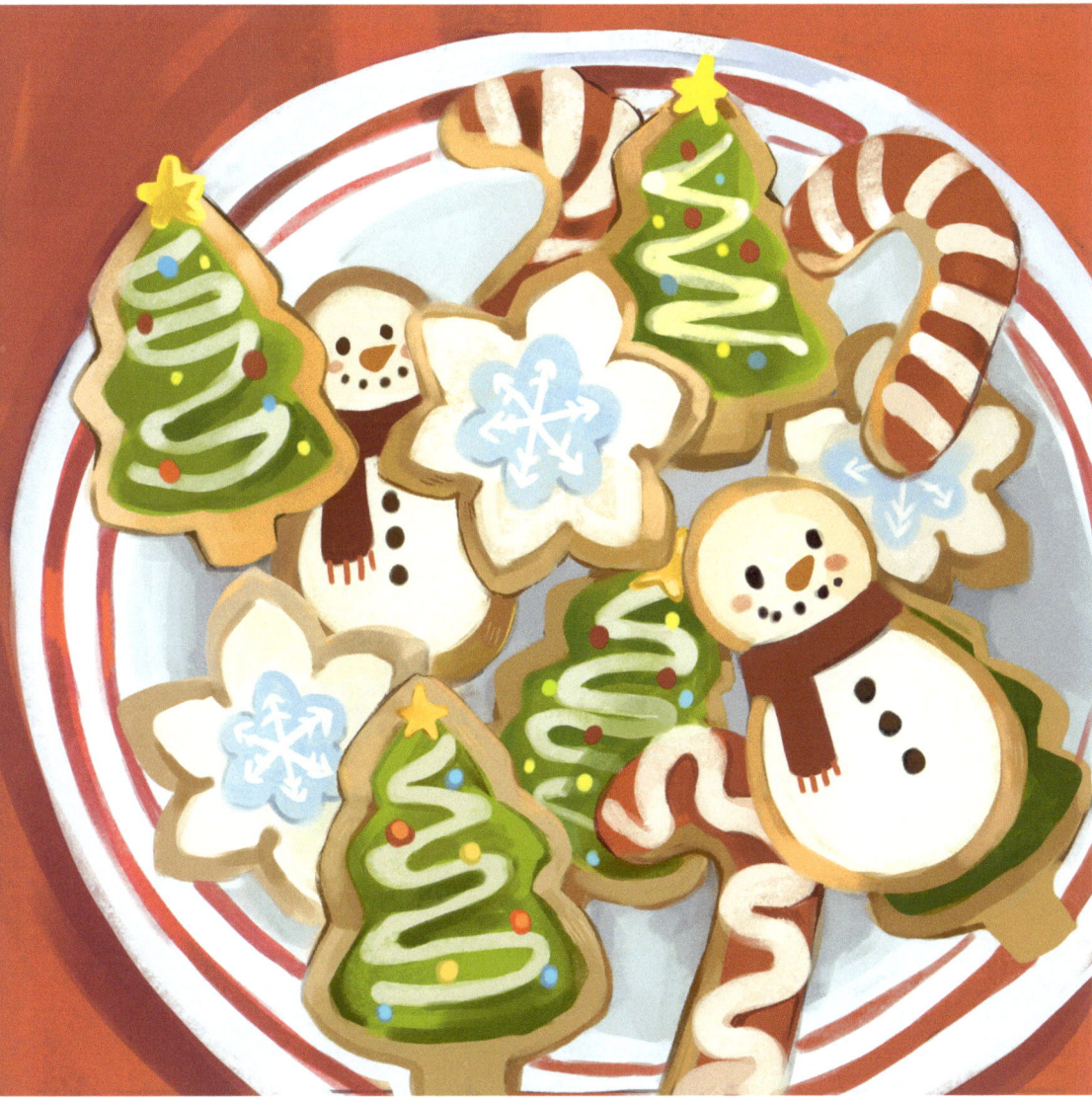

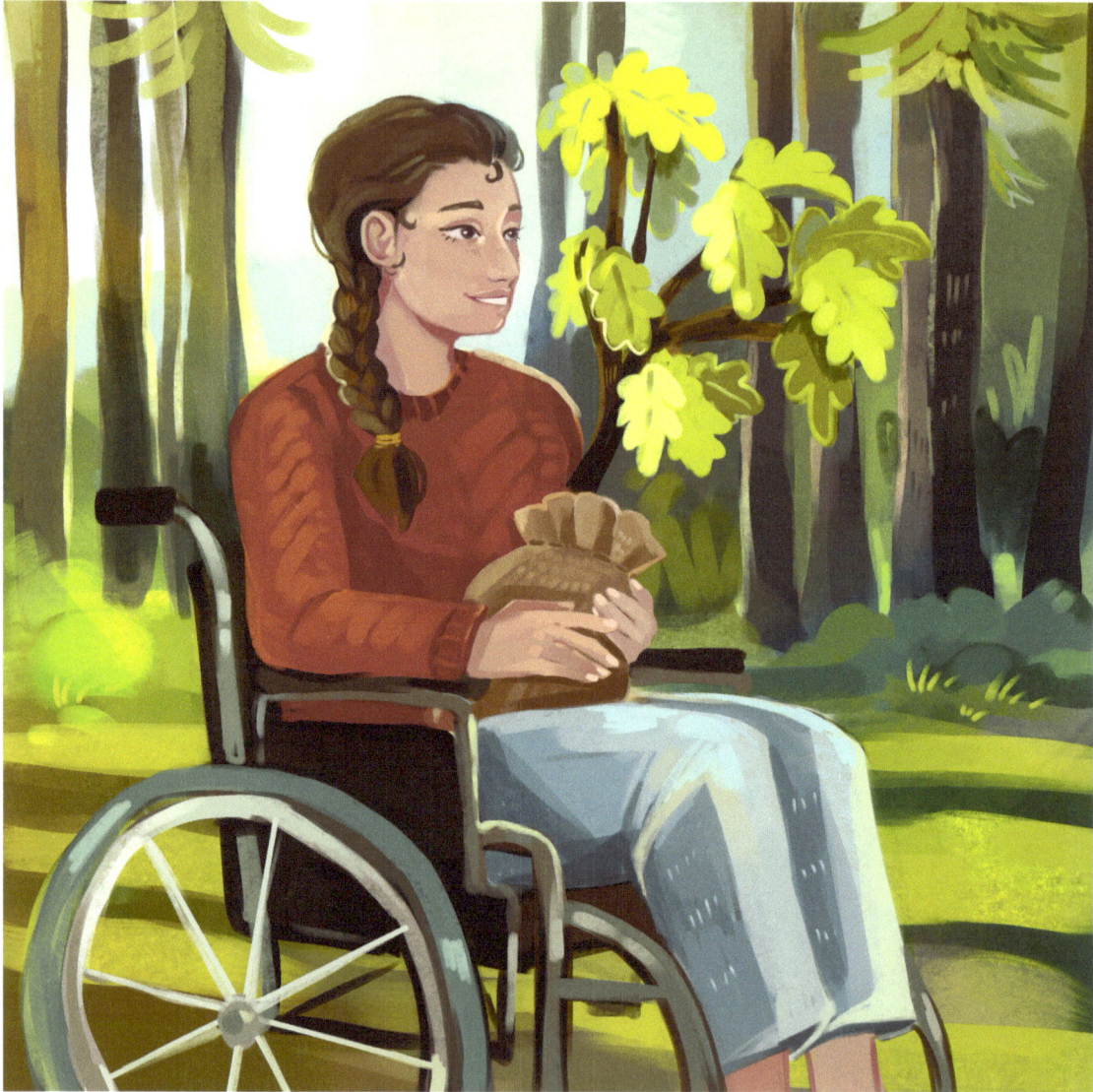

16

Volunteer in the community

One dearly-departed gal pal and I met volunteering for Trees Atlanta. She would photograph our events for the organization, and occasionally help us to plant, mulch, and prune trees around the city. We would only see each other on those days, but with our hands in the dirt, we would talk about what was going on in our lives. We bonded over a love of nature and trees! When you volunteer, you can make new friends or strengthen the connection with your current ones—all while doing something impactful for your community.

17

Bring out their favorite libation

In Texas, there's no shortage of margarita varieties: fruit flavored, "skinny," "virgin," frozen, on the rocks, and so on. When I see that blue-rimmed margarita glass, I often think of my mom, who would drink these with friends (or my dad) while eating Mexican food. When you're meeting your friend out and you know their libation of choice, bring it or order it for them. It's a nice way to set the tone for the time together and it makes them feel appreciated! As an extra, have a special glass ready for them (maybe with their name on it, like a girlfriend did for me).

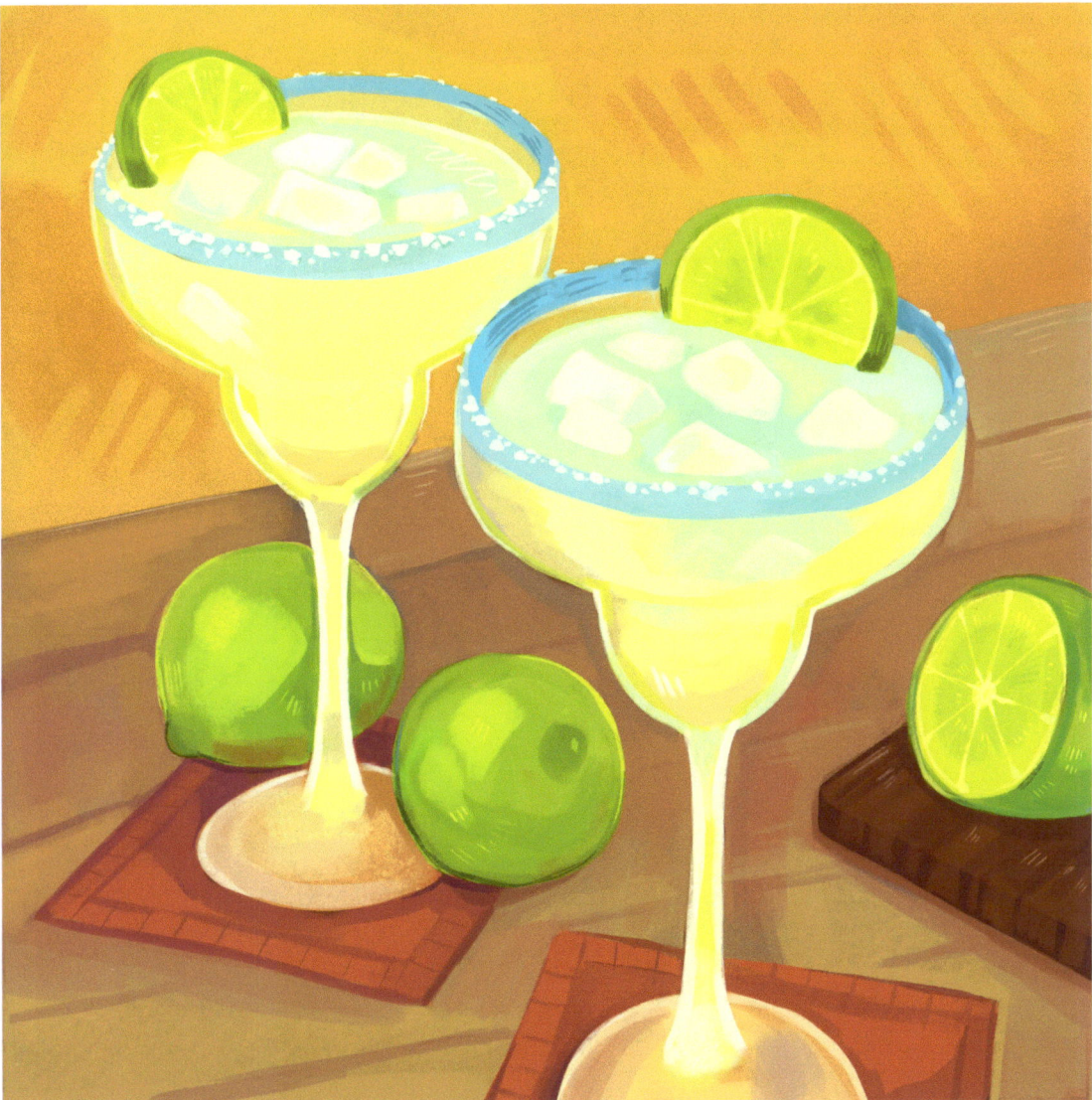

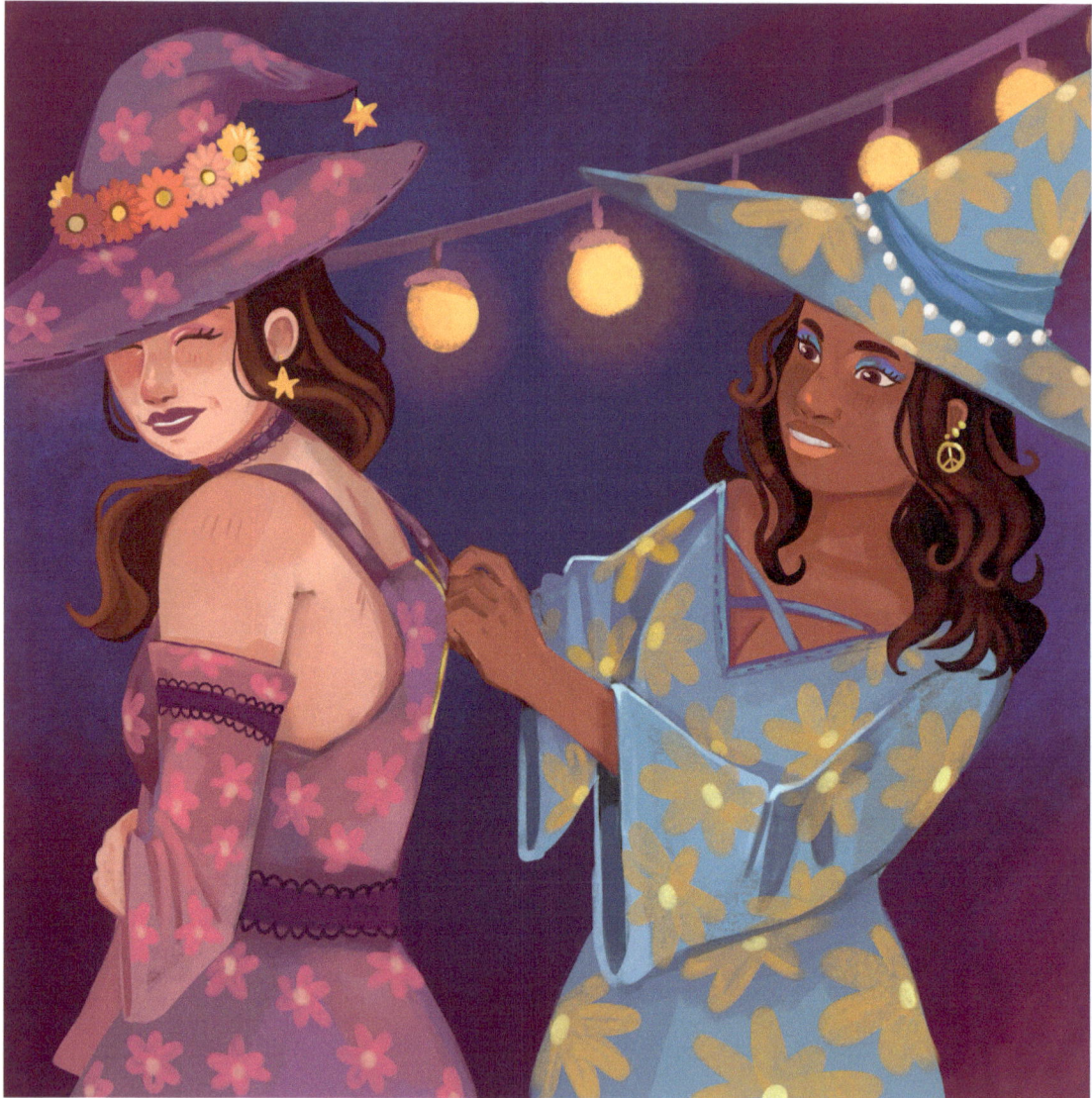

18

Play dressup

Do you remember your first adult costume party? Or your most recent one? A newly-engaged woman I knew was invited to her husband-to-be's big work Halloween event. It was her first one with him, and she was uncertain about what costume to wear, how creative to be, and how much glitz to add. She wanted to be festive, but not too festive; garnering attention but not overly so. In a smart move, she invited a new acquaintance over—one who knew her fiancé and had been to the event in prior years—to test out some combinations. Together, they created a look that inspired confidence. Sharing an experience like that is often the beginning of a long-lasting friendship.

19

Respond to important emails together

"It's your first chance to show them how you negotiate," I answered when my friend asked me what I thought of the emailed offer letter to her new job opportunity. She was excited about the job but was surprised at the base salary. Was she expecting too much? How should she respond? In situations like these, it's good to bounce ideas off a friend. In her case, we knew she would be negotiating contracts on a regular basis so we brainstormed the best way to approach it. We composed the email, anticipating their various responses. She got the role—and the salary—she wanted!

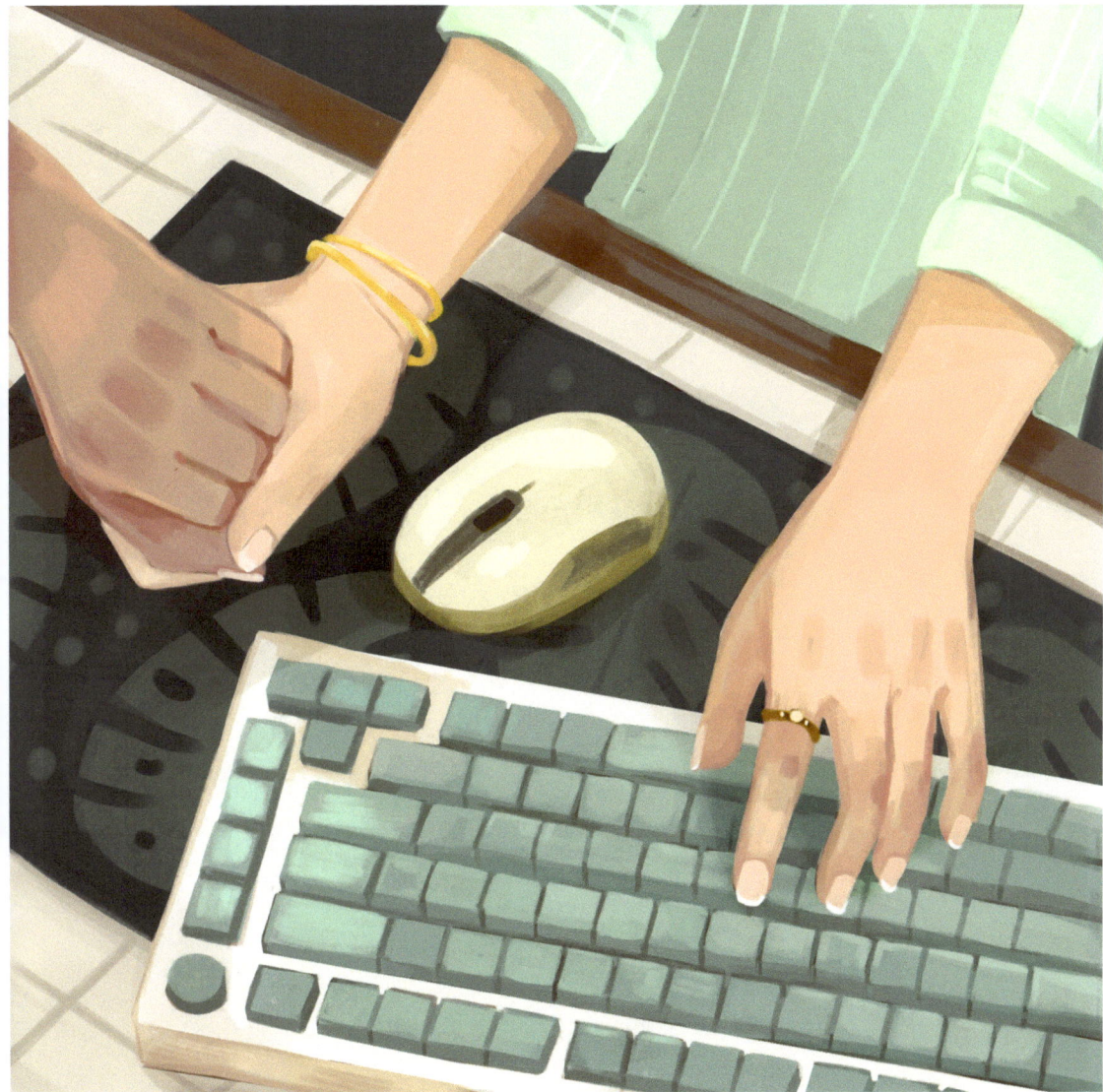

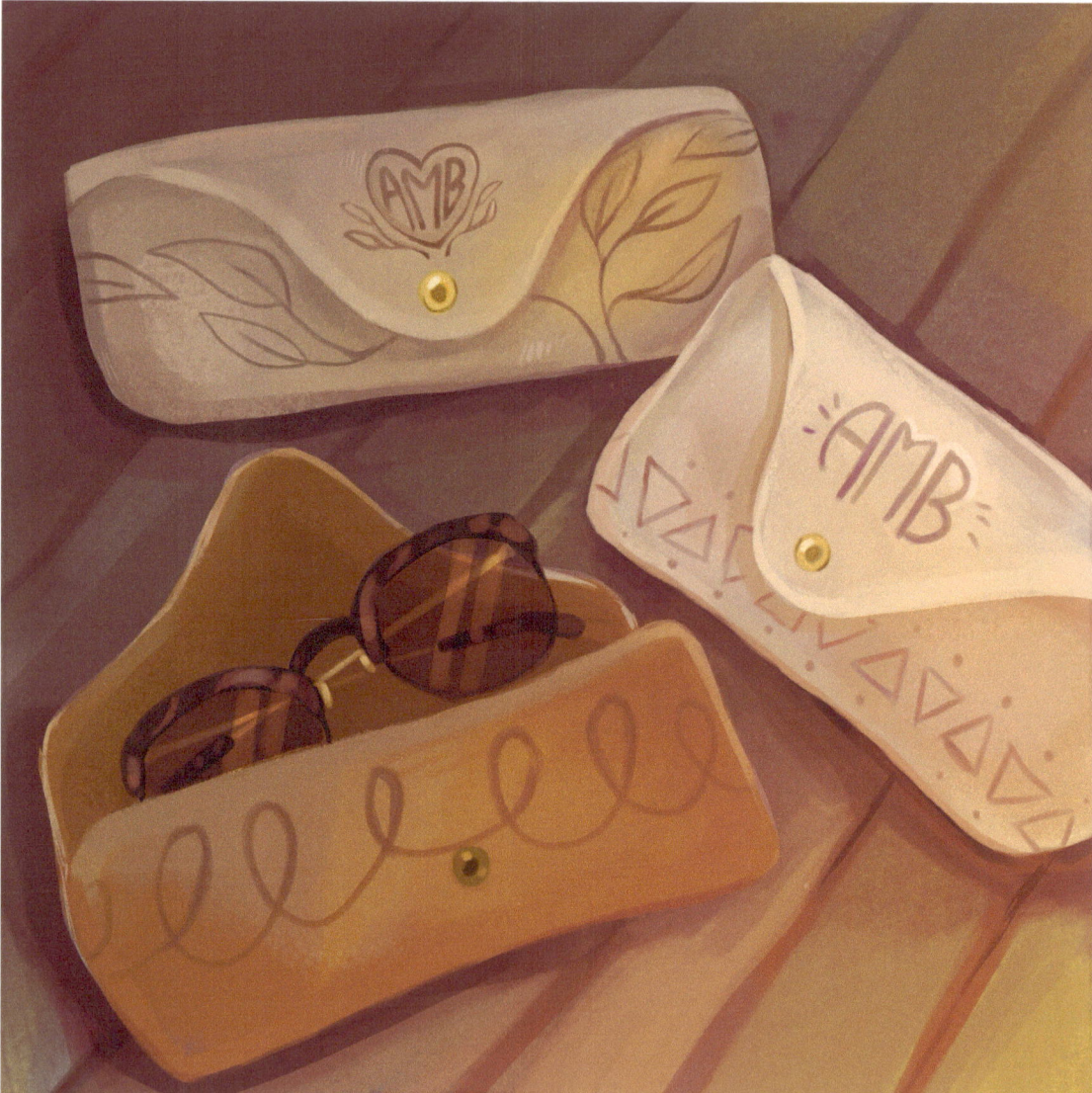

20

Personalize a "just because" gift

Recently, someone said to me how much she wanted a Cricut® craft machine to personalize her child's wardrobe. Adding a name to your belongings gives it extra meaning because it's all yours, and not meant for anyone else. Adding a name or monogram to a handcrafted gift is deeply personal, especially when there's no obligatory time to give it. Those presents—made by hand and personalized, that are also "just what I wanted!"—will be treasured, because the recipient knows what went into creating them.

21
Sing your favorite songs

High school, college, and post-college single-days memories often include songs we have sung together, perfectly in harmony or drunkenly off-key. Songs from movies, concerts, beaches, bars, or dances, especially with catchy refrains, form the soundtracks of our lives. As we get older, those songs can carry special memories of being with friends and belting out those tunes. These days, I'll find myself on the phone with far-away pals singing, "Tell Me More, Tell Me More," "Walking on Sunshine" or "STOP, In the Name of Love." It's like time and distance between us have evaporated.

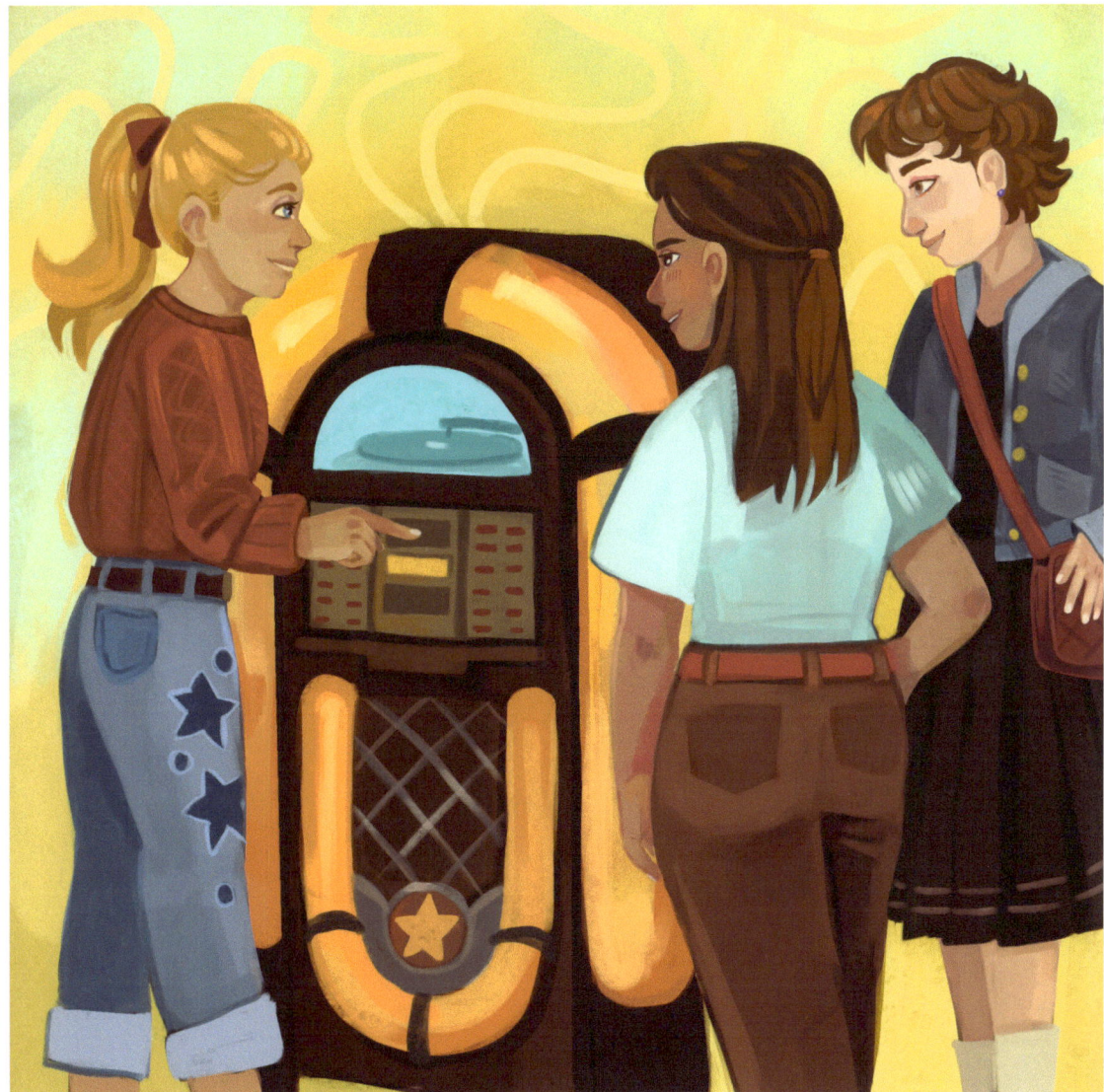

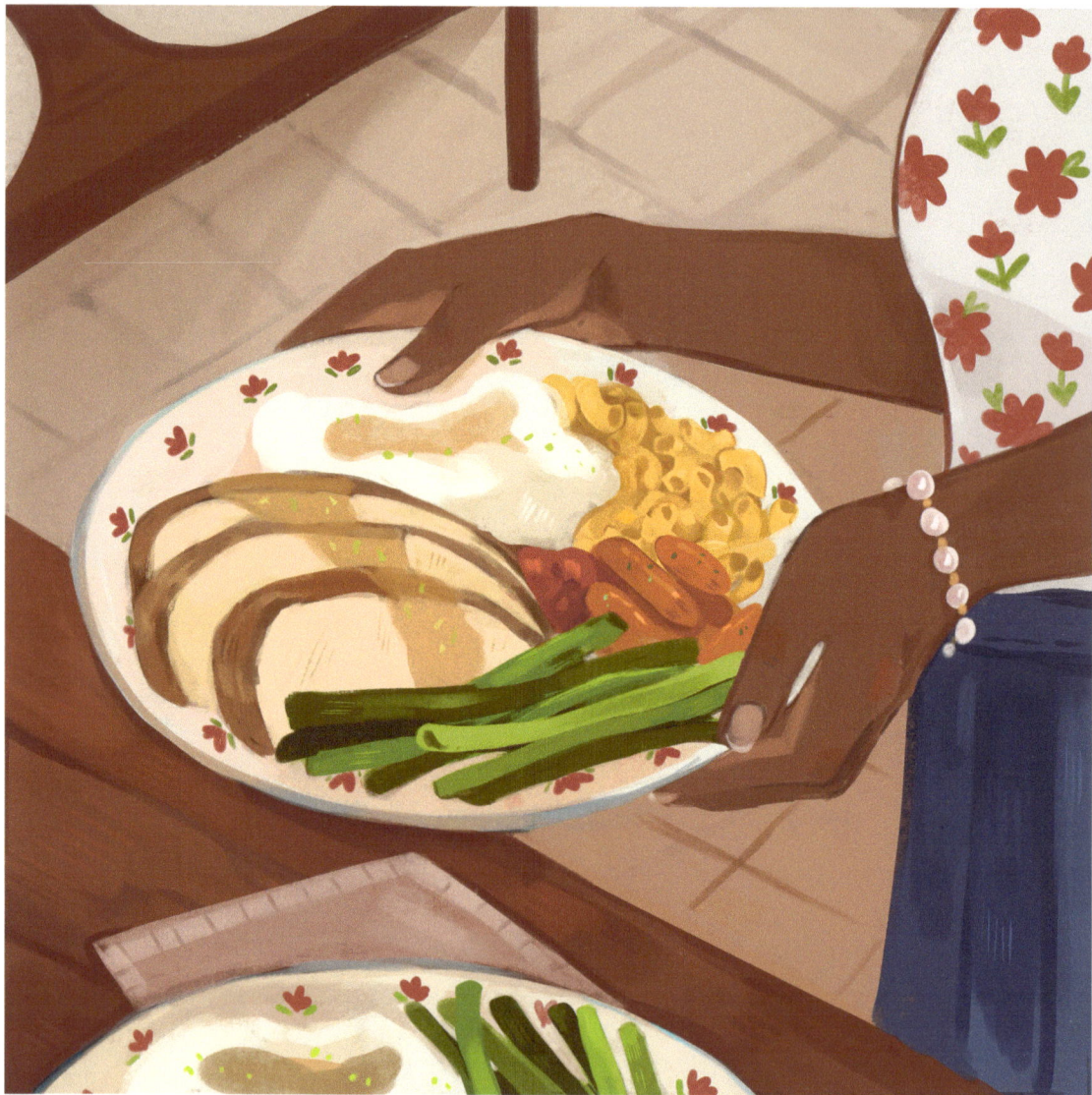

22

Play chef or sous chef

My neighbor panicked when she heard that her in-laws planned on eating Thanksgiving at her house! She had never hosted a holiday home-cooked meal. She asked me for suggestions on the menu, cooking cadence, and table prep. Then she asked for my help in the kitchen, which I was glad to do. After she'd decided what was going to be done, we divvied up the work and I did what she needed graciously. Remember, you can make suggestions till the cows come home, but whoever owns the kitchen is in charge! You want to avoid any hurt feelings by taking over—and you'll want to stay friends afterwards.

23

Share home care resources

Home warranty-approved contractors, repair apps, and social media are rife with suggestions (many of them good), but nothing beats the recommendations of a friend you know and trust. Having a go-to person for a specific job (like a handyman or plumber), or narrowing the many choices to two or three to get bids is so valuable. Our realtor has become my BFF not only for her expertise in the real estate industry, but also for possible resources to address home problems. Now that I've begun my own contractor list, I'll be glad to share the names of these talented professionals with any who ask me.

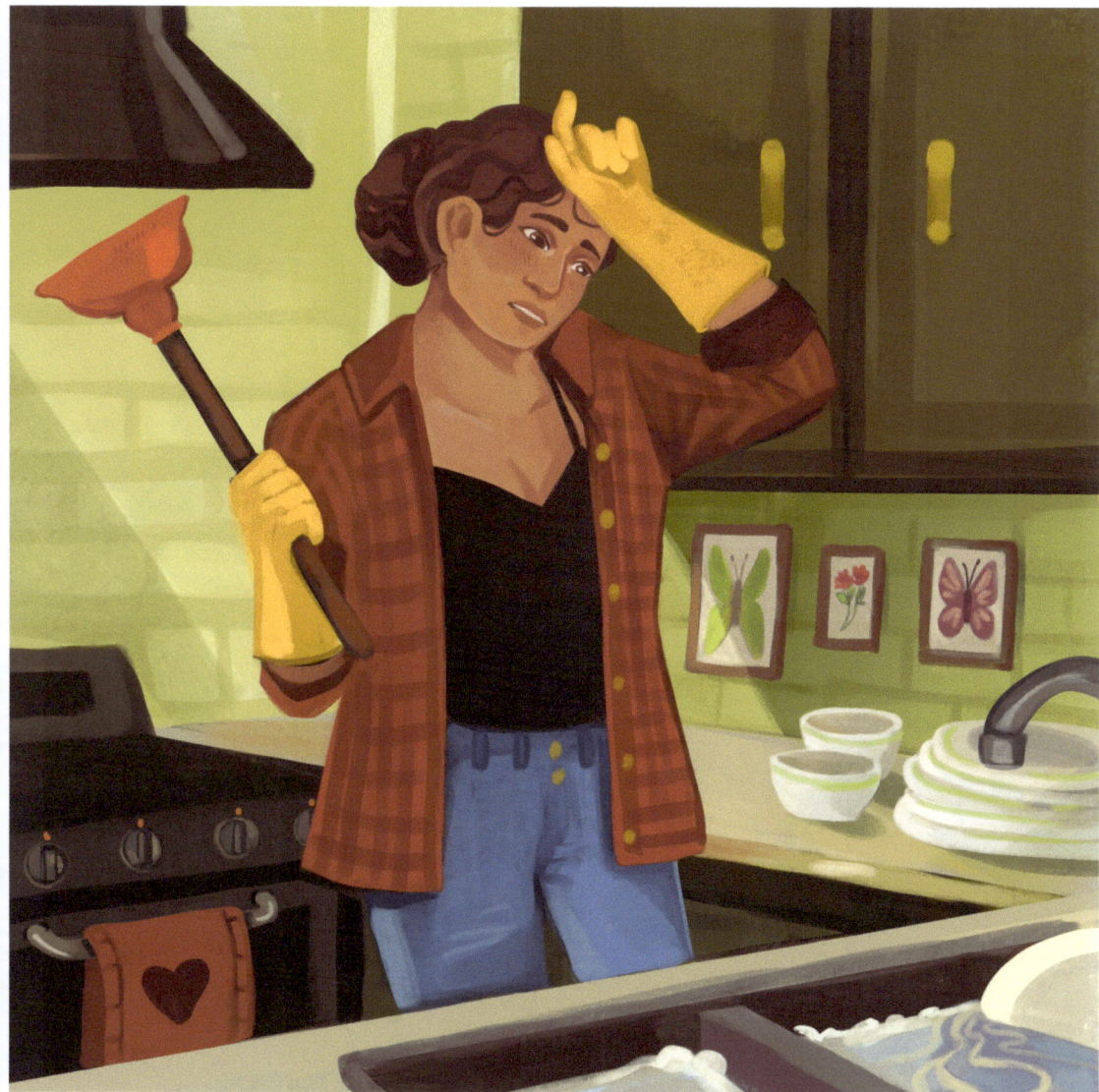

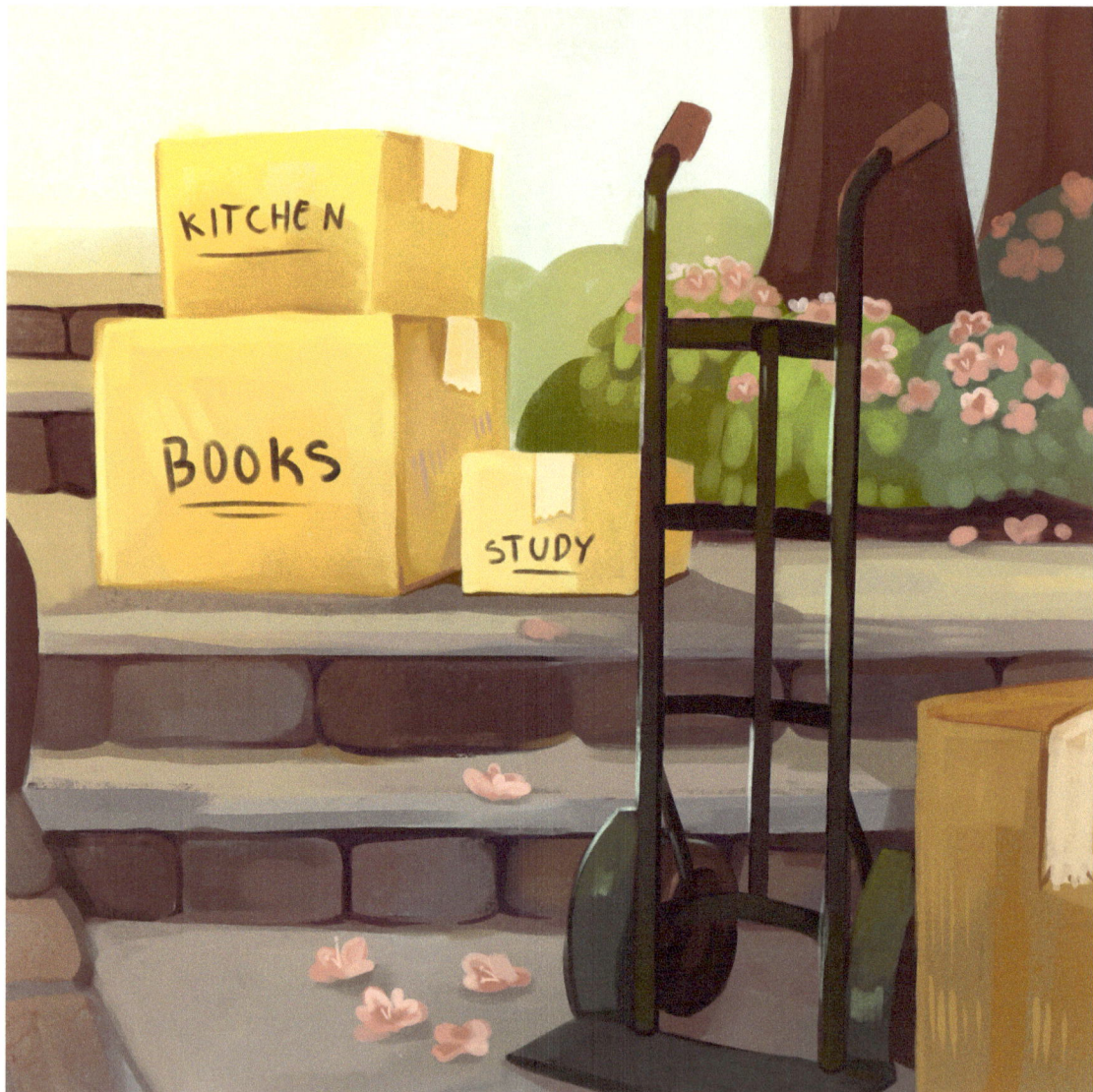

24

Help with moving day

In college, moving usually happened twice a year. It was exhausting but very social, and I can remember being excited about change and laughing a lot. These days, moving doesn't happen as often. It is still exhausting, and often difficult or sad—especially when we're leaving loved ones behind. Friends can help on Moving Day or packing days beforehand, like filling boxes with precious, hand-carry items. On the flip side, if you're a friend helping someone getting acclimated to a new place, helping them unpack can be a special time. Those first few days in a new home is a great time to make new memories.

25

Tear up with them

One of my most cherished memories is a small ceremony that my very dear Georgian friend had for me after a tragic personal loss. That day, she met me at sunrise near a lake with prayers and a small meal. She encouraged me to cry, talk, or be silent—whatever I needed to help heal and move forward. She was THERE, and I am forever grateful to her. While I don't wish tragedy on anyone, I do wish everyone to have a gal pal to cry with—whether that's at the movies, at sad news, at joyful news, or with belly-hurting laughter.

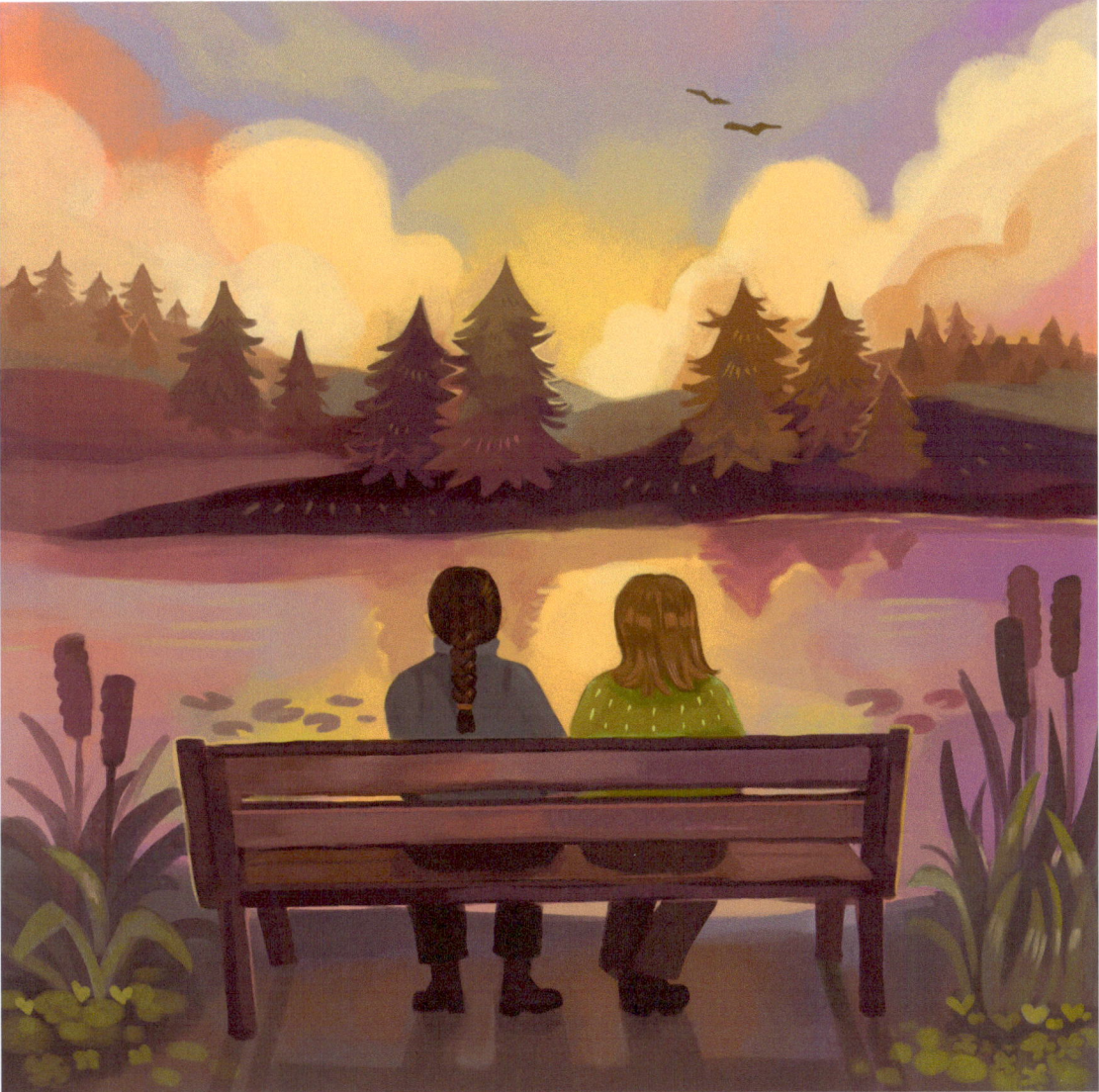

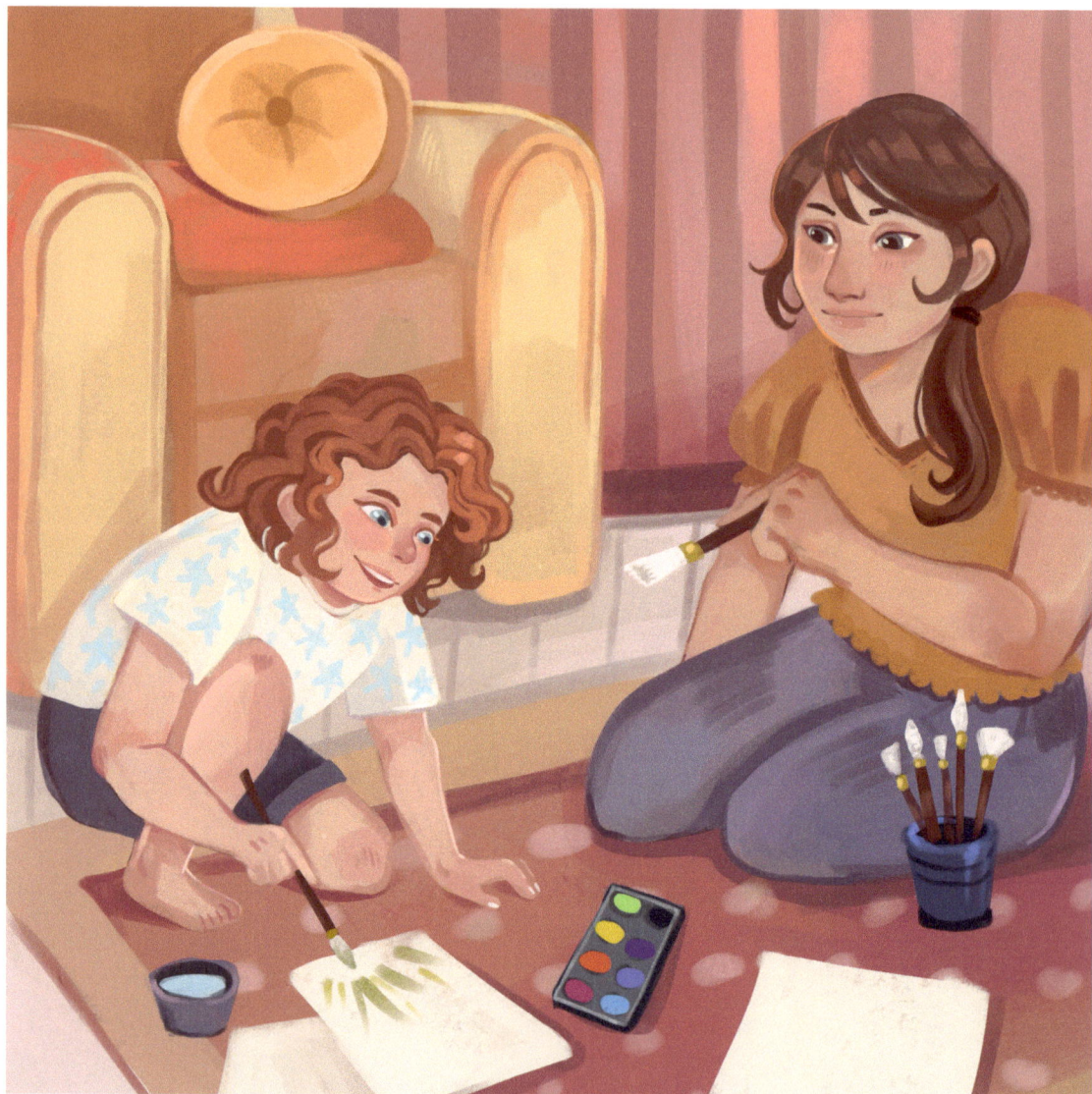

26

Kid-sit when they need a break

A colleague of my husband was blessed with three children under five. He and his wife wanted, and needed, an occasional break caring for them. Their mom, an energetic and creative person, assembled grandparents, friends, and neighbors as a little care task force—especially when the boys were small—to kid-sit them or take them for visits while she and her husband had a little "alone time." Watching small children is not for everyone, but most people can help kid-sit if there are just one or two little munchkins to watch.

27

Test perfumes, spices, or teas

They say the olfactory sense (smelling) is the second sense to develop (after hearing). Evolutionarily, it has been the one that helps us determine what foods to eat and protects us from poison. In our modern days, we also know it is part of the chemistry of attraction and relaxation. A certified aromatherapist and tea vendor taught me about how fragrance can help to immerse yourself in different, dreamy environments. Go with a friend into a spice and tea shop, or go to a fragrance counter to try different fragrances together! You'll see that you're naturally attracted to some and repelled by others as you discover new worlds through aromas.

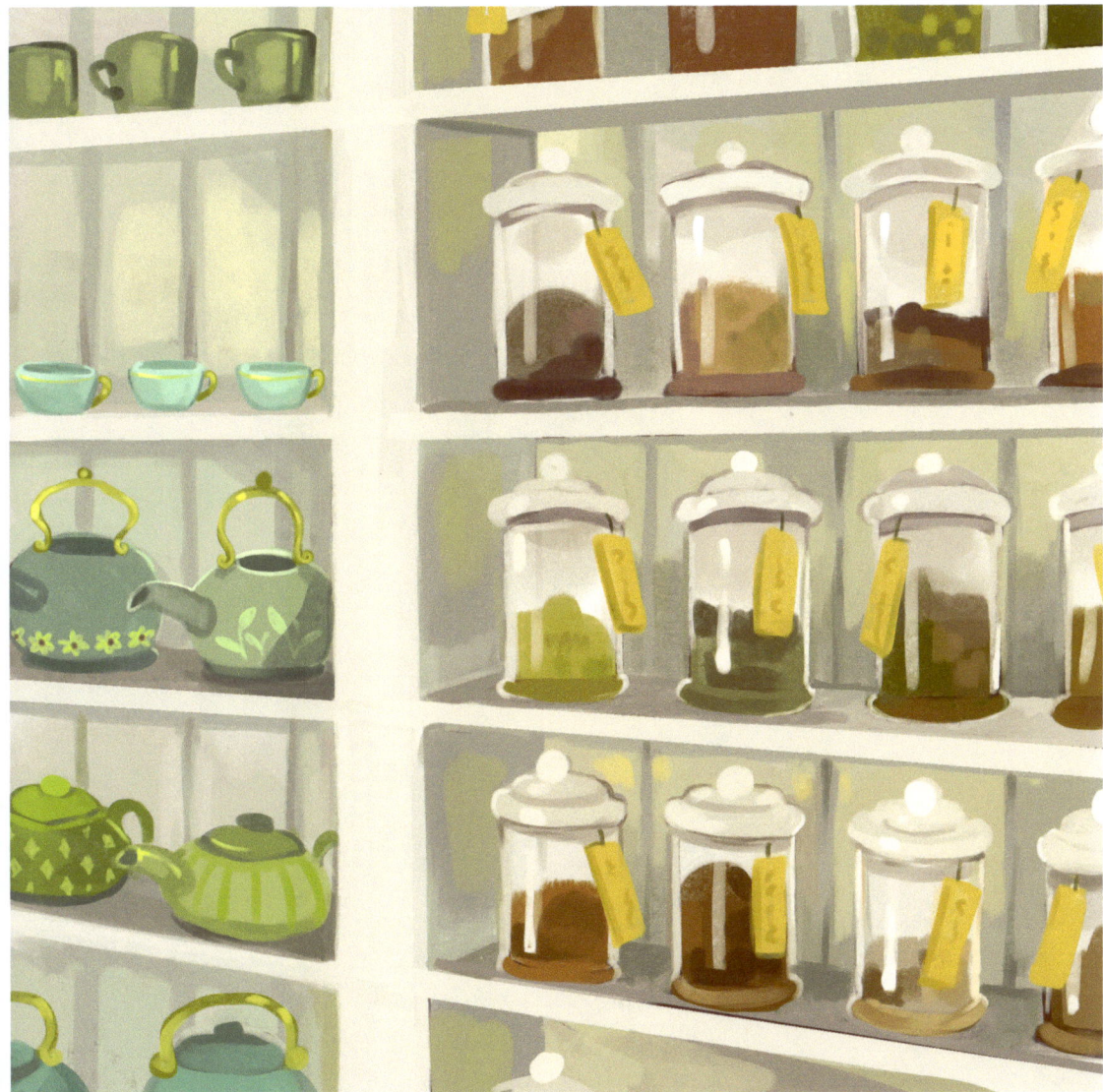

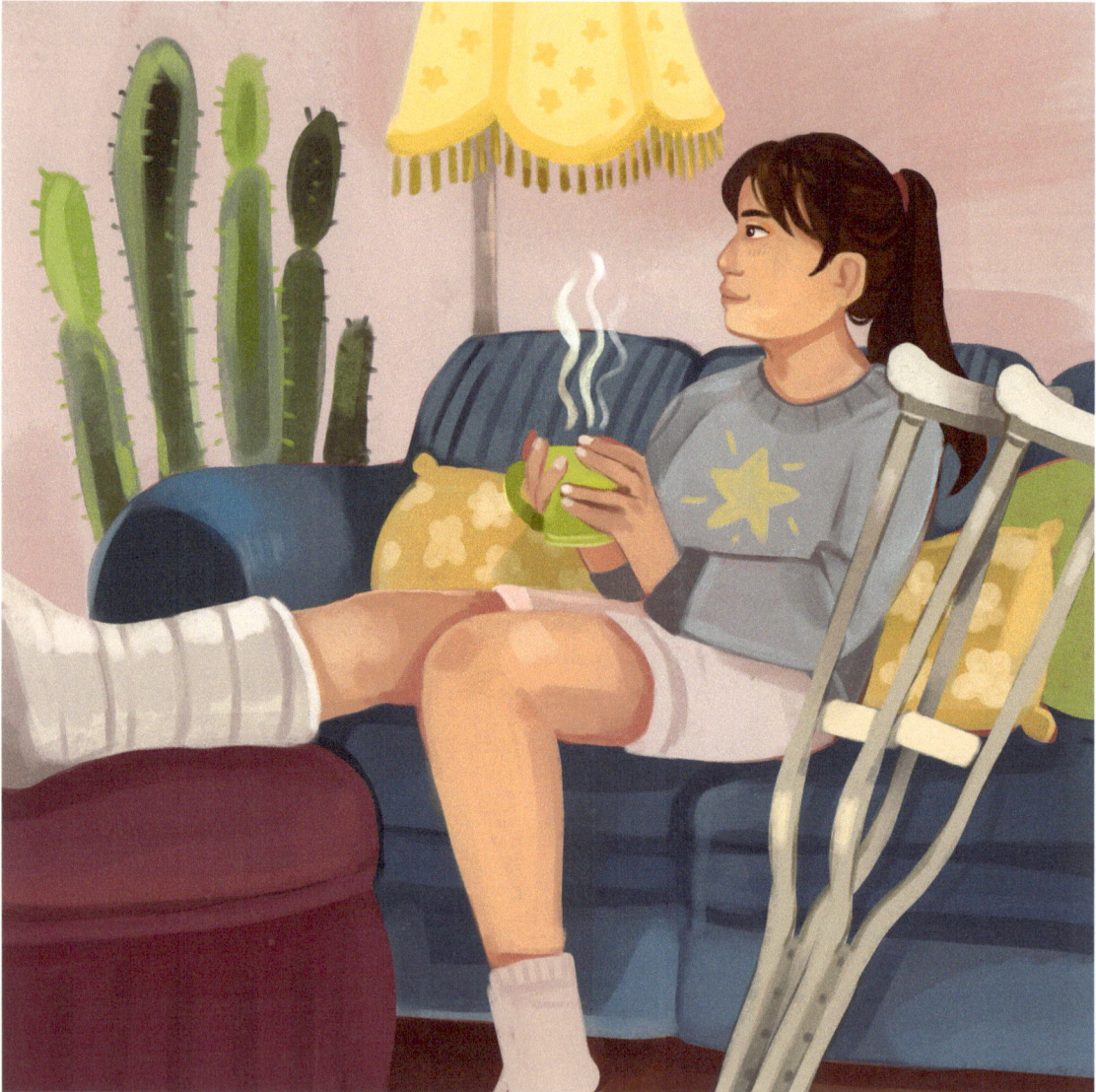

28

Assist when they're injured

It's a real friend that will help you when you're physically hurt, especially if you need crutches, a sling, or a walker (and I've needed all three). When a friend is hurt, listen to what she says she needs, and try to anticipate what she *really* needs. You may be able to go one step better! Like when I hurt my shoulder and one friend helped me put boxes in my car, or when my best friend ever—my husband—washed and even styled my hair during the first two weeks after surgery. Priceless! Remember to assist lovingly, and don't hold it against her later.

29

Join a book club together

If you both like to read, read together. . . and join others who do as well! In a group, you can really enjoy analyzing a business book, tackling a fitness tome, escaping into historical fiction, or sailing through an easy beach read. Recently-published books will often have Book Club Questions at the back to help you discuss plots, characters, methods, settings, and alternative actions. The wider variety of people that you attract to your book club circle, the wider range of opinions and interpretations! Be sure to let everyone speak their minds without judgments, to keep those conversations lively and enjoyable.

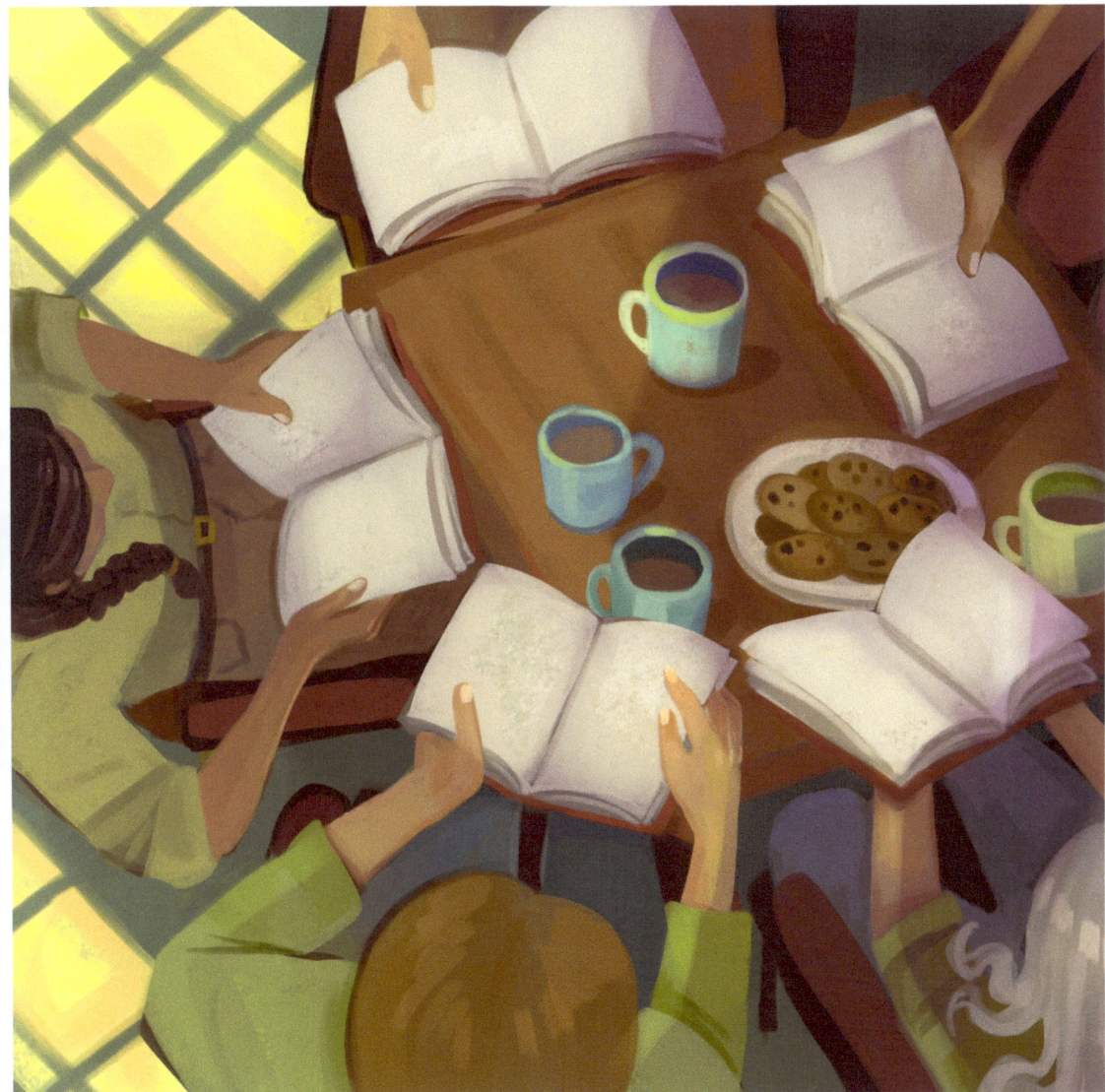

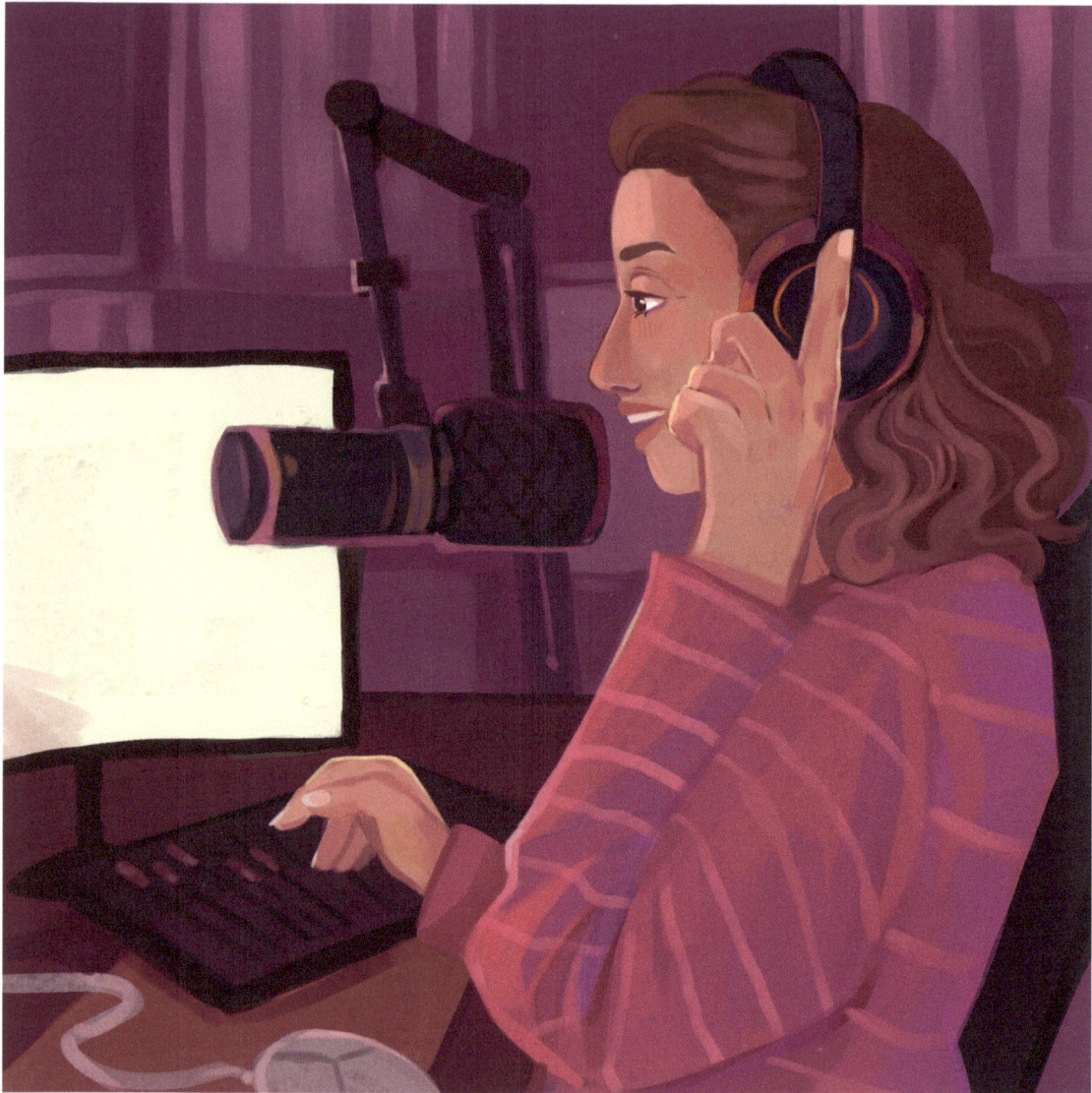

30

Make a radio station shout out

Have you ever wanted to contact a radio station to dedicate a song or give a shout out? It's easier than ever through their digital channels. If you know that your friend will be listening to her favorite station on her special day, write out a special message for her. Gather up some courage and make the effort to contact the station. Text her to make sure she's listening when it is due to be broadcast, and then record the on-air announcement on your phone when it happens. After, you can send it to her so that she has it to listen to again and again.

31

Go to the doctor with her—and keep it private

As I said in *Stoplights Are For Kissing*, The "White Coat Syndrome" is well documented: people get nervous in front of medical professionals. If she asks you to go to a particularly scary appointment, make every effort to go with her. Ask her ahead of time if she'd like you to participate or be quiet, but either way, keep close to her. Pay attention and take notes to make sure you remember the doctor's comments right. Then, get a phone number or email of someone to call with questions later. Remember that healthcare issues are private, and don't discuss what happened in that office with anyone but her.

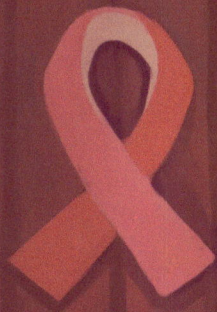

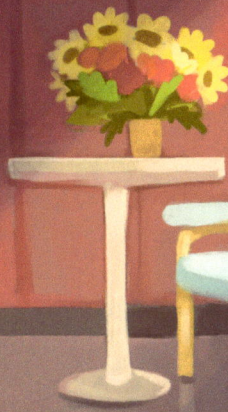

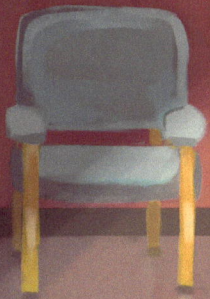

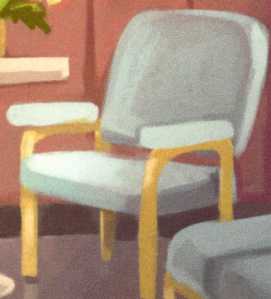

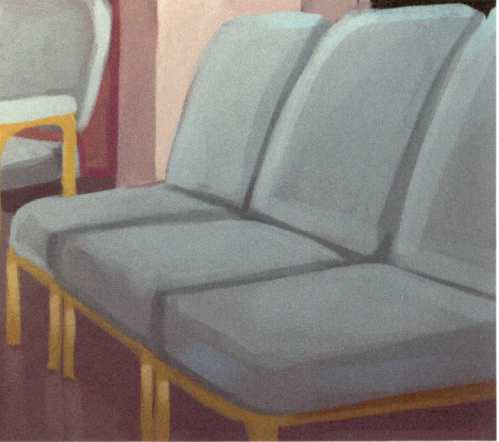

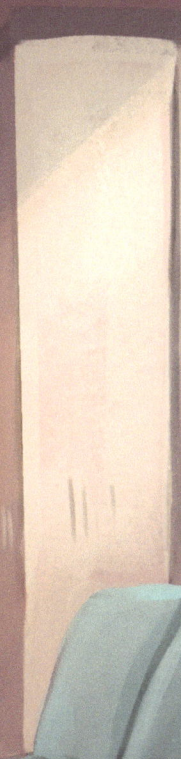

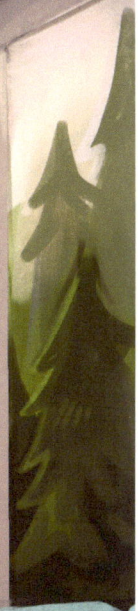

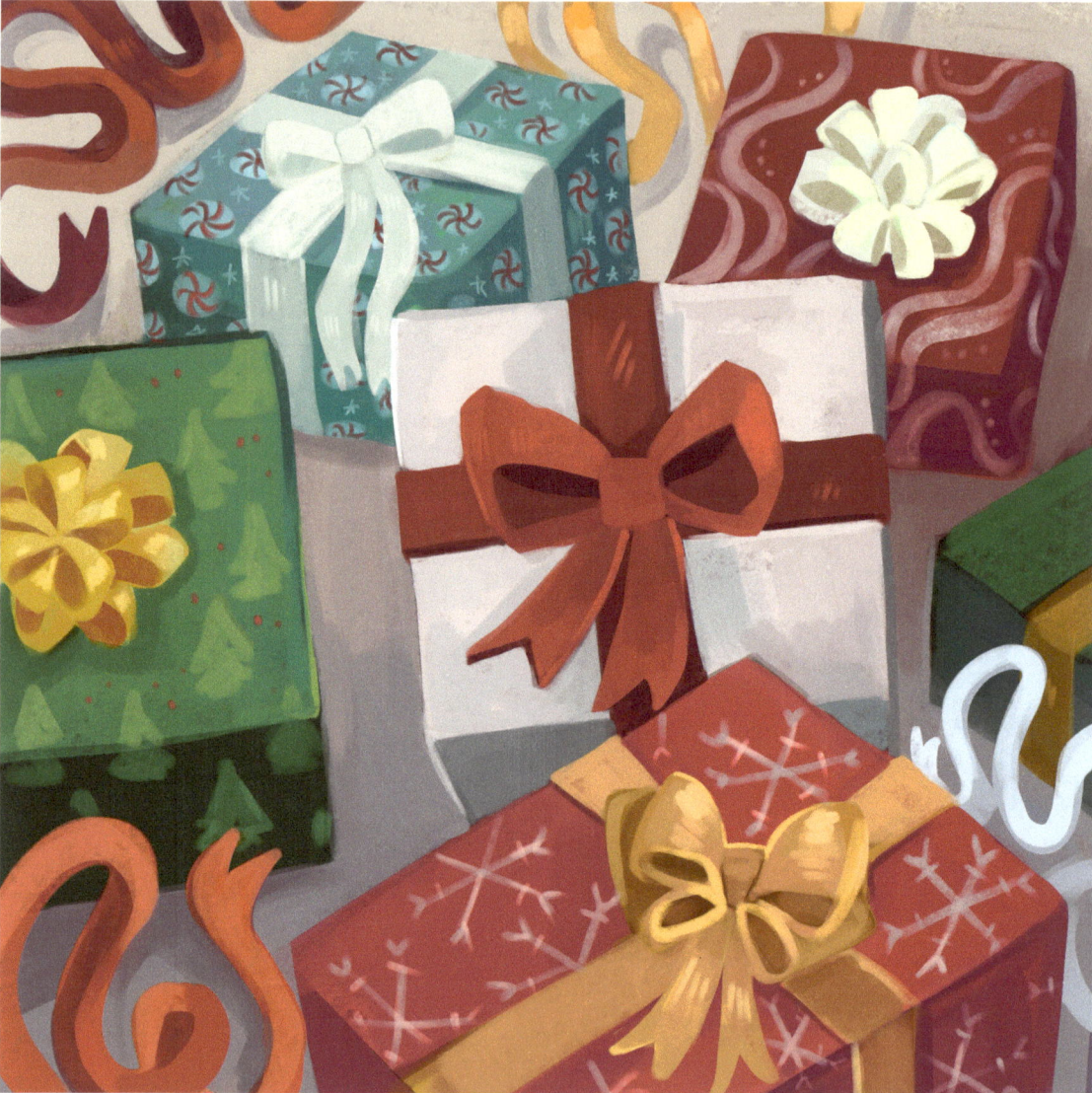

32

Wrap it up

An older woman in my life loved to wrap presents. She had worked in the gift wrap department of a store and learned the finer points of elegant presentations: perfect corners, matching patterns, hidden tape, curling ribbon, and an ornamented bow. She taught me a trick or two when we would wrap gifts for the holidays. These days, I love to have a wrapping party with holiday music, hot cocoa and tons of supplies to make each gift look different. Hauling the presents and supplies to one location is a bit of a challenge that can be overcome with a grocery cart or wagon—and the final products are worth it!

33

Refer financial professionals

Navigating the spheres of money can be daunting; estate planning, investments, taxes, legal issues, insurance, and banking are all disciplines in their own rights. While prior generations of women usually didn't manage these areas, it's more common in the SHEconomy for us to do so. Building your network of key advisors is an important step in understanding your financial position. Trusted investment bankers, attorneys, financial planners, and insurance agents should be shared, so don't be shy about asking for recommendations from others. In those professions, most business development is by word of mouth.

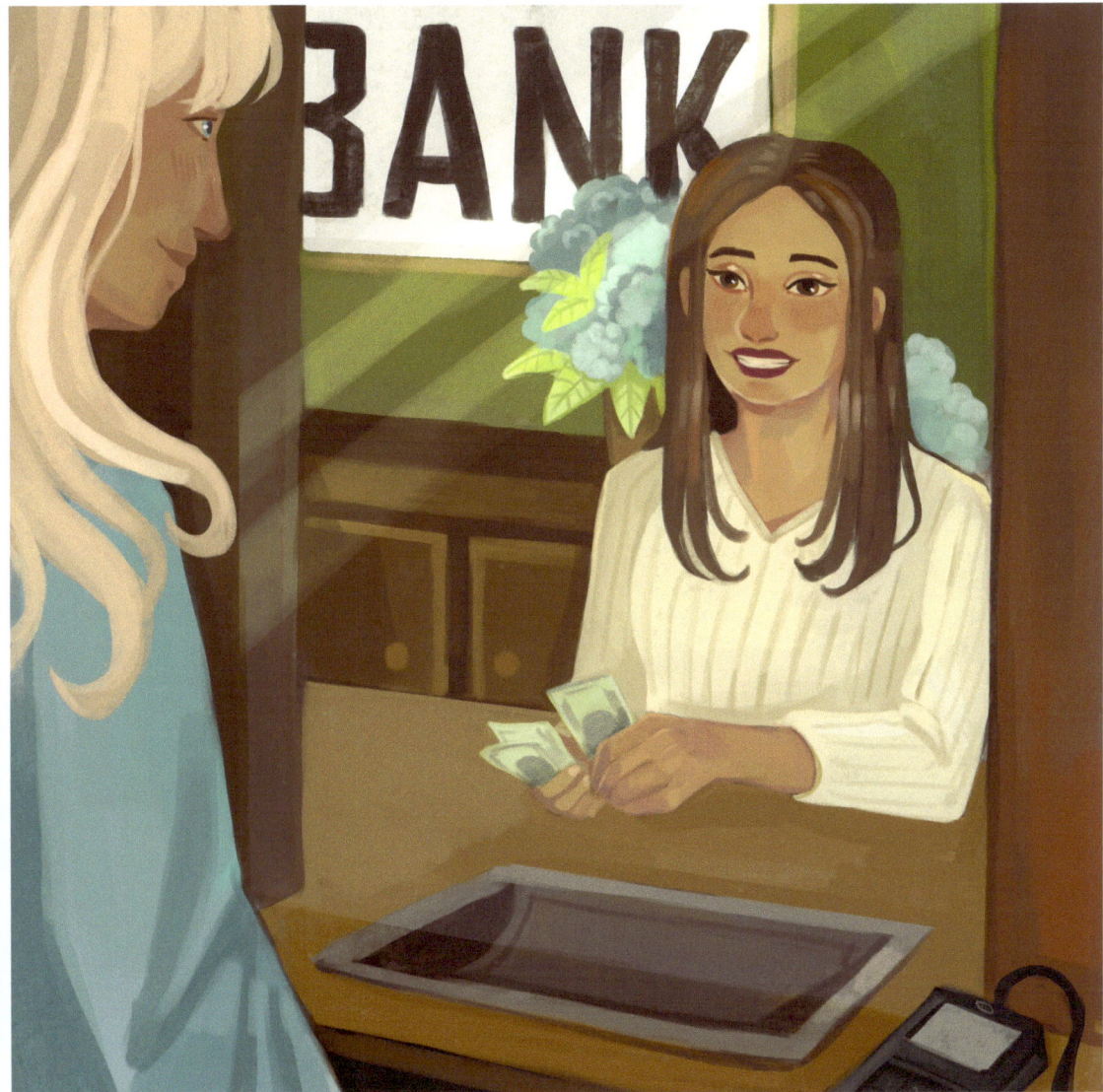

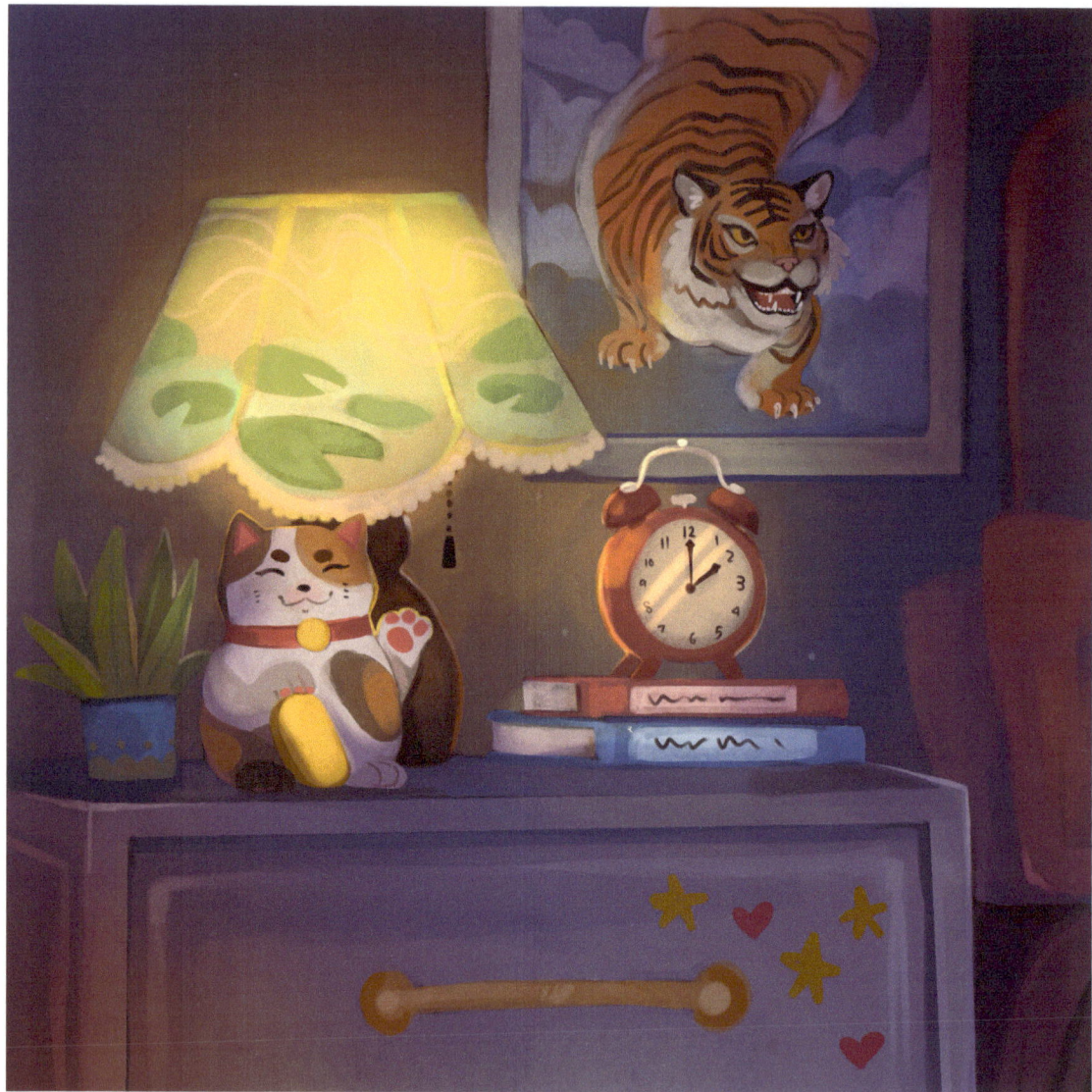

34

Don't send it to voicemail

No good news comes after midnight, unless you're expecting a baby. The snooze and Do Not Disturb functions on our phones are there to help us have fewer interruptions as we sleep. No matter how tired you are or how important the next morning's events are, your dear friends and family will thank you if you pick up the phone when there is an emergency. Most of us only have a few of these people in our lives, so set your phone to take their calls no matter what time they come in—and ask them to do the same for you.

35

Recommend them as speakers

Earning recognition through speaking is a good career builder and business development tool. Professional conferences, academic panels, networking groups, and podcasts routinely need qualified speakers for their events. If you're asked to participate but have a conflict or no interest, look at it as an opportunity to do two nice things: recommend a friend in your industry to get the exposure and assist the organizers in filling the slot. It makes good sense to keep a list of people you can cross-connect for these engagements (then let them know you'd like to be considered in their recommendations as well).

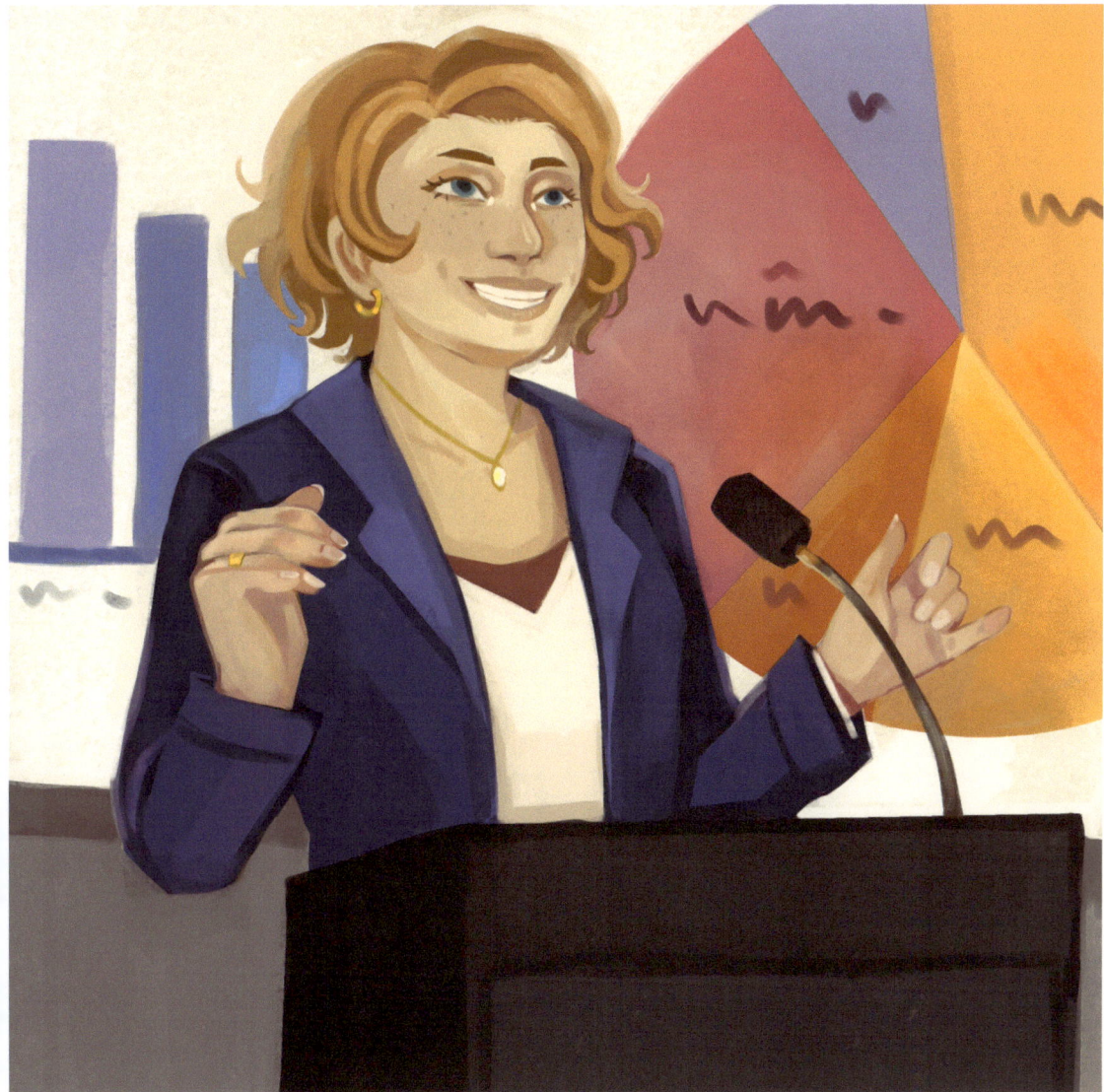

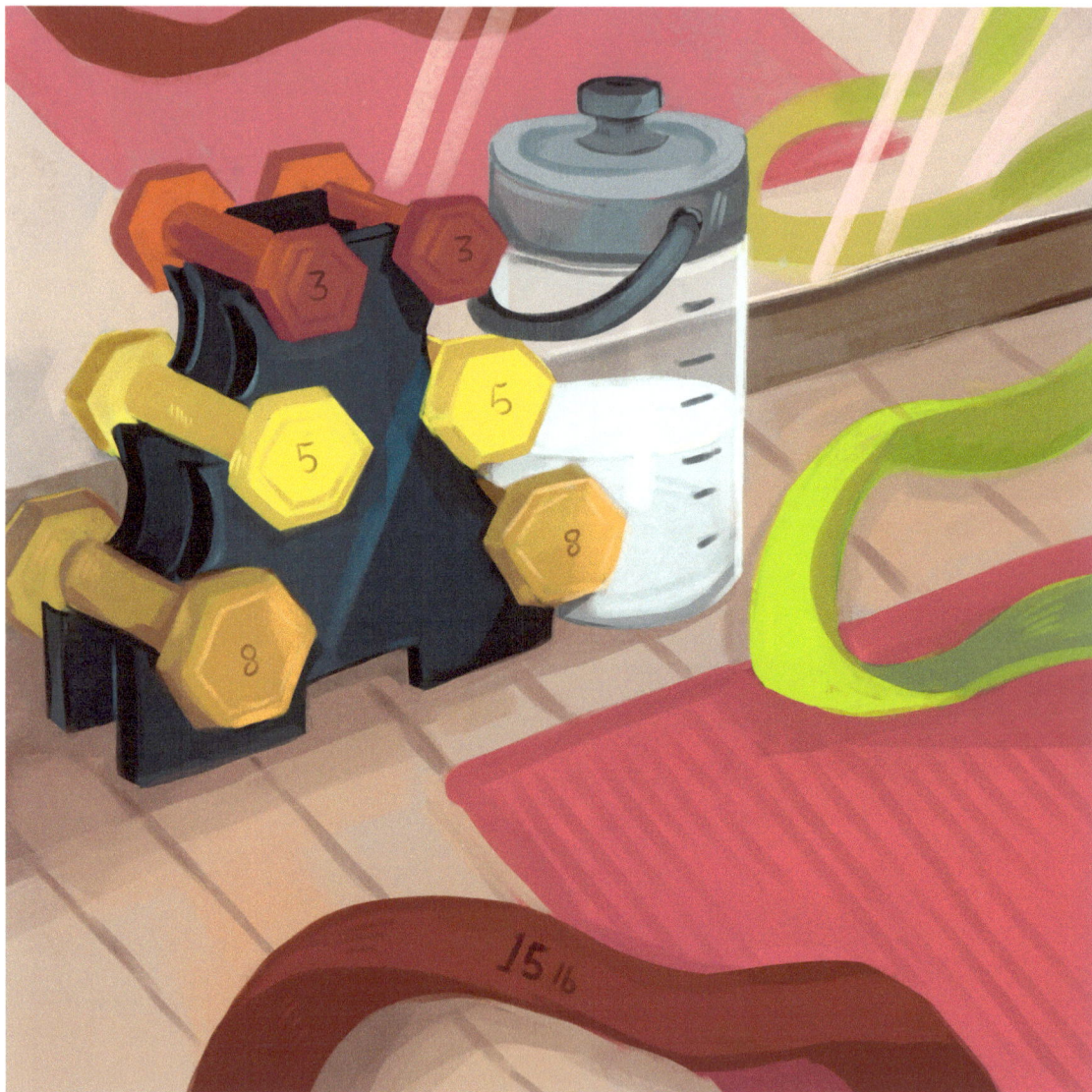

36

Be a workout accountability partner

Not everyone can be in the JacFit 5am club (and not everyone wants to be), yet most of us like a clean bill of health. Unfortunately, that doesn't happen by itself, so teaming up with a pal that has similar fitness goals helps immeasurably. When I agreed to a 30-mile walk to benefit breast cancer research, thank goodness a woman who had done it before (25 years older than me) agreed to let me train with her. I kept at it because of her—no question about it—and was able to complete it. We became friends after those training walks, though my days of long-distance walking are probably over.

37

Stretch to do a new sport or hobby

If you've ever seen the movie "The Intern," you may remember the scene where Robert DeNiro's character introduces his boss, played by Anne Hathaway, to tai chi. He learned the martial art after his wife died, she needed a way to relax. We're never too old or advanced in our career to try something new. Find someone experienced and go together for your first few tries. If you'd like to try golfing, for example, you may want to share a cart and a caddy with someone who knows the course and the rules of the game. The same can be said about pickleball—have fun learning.

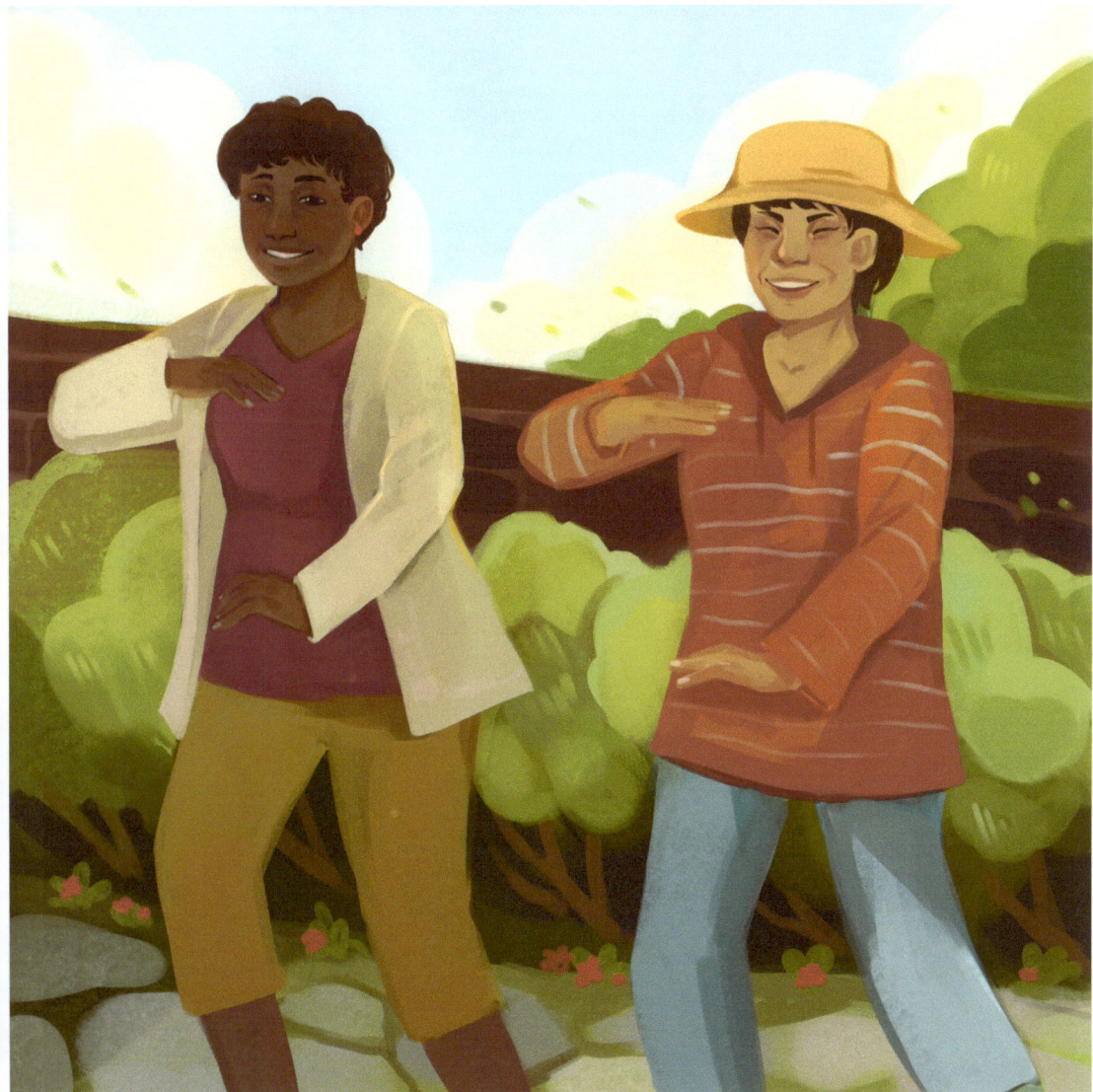

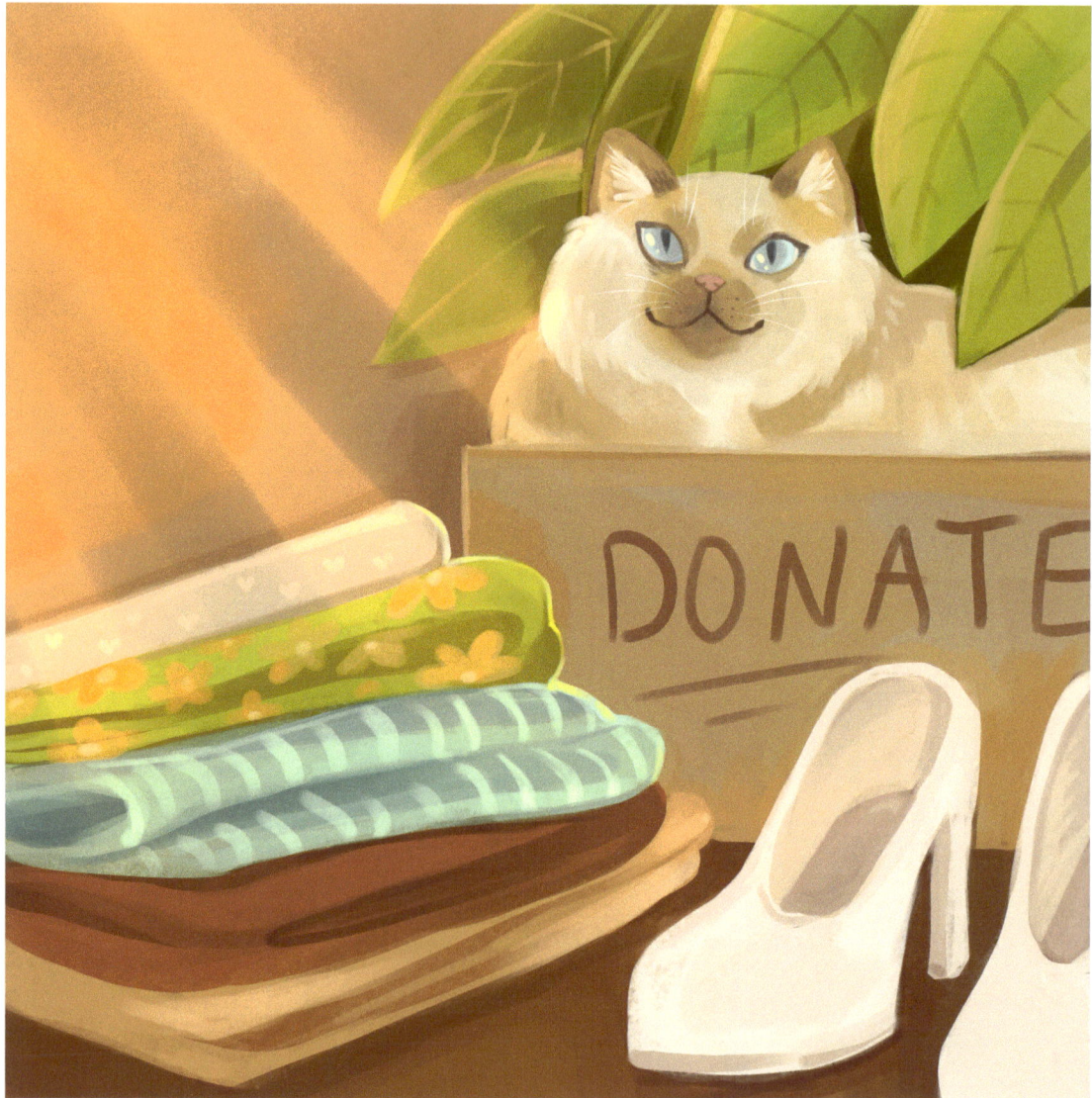
DONATE

38

Play "what not to wear"

Not all of us have a friend who is a professional organizer or stylist, but most of us have a friend who will tell us if what we're wearing flatters us or not. It's easy to hold on to pieces that used to fit us (but don't now), or accessories we never wear (that purse was expensive!), or well-worn goodies (in fashion 10 years ago). Like hairstyles, fashion changes, and our clothing should fit us and reflect our lifestyles as we age. Ask a trusted friend to review your closet, decide what to donate, or have a swap event between closets of others about the same size.

39

Belly-laugh

One of the best parts of having a sister-who-is-also-a-friend is the shared history of growing up. When we see each other or talk online, we catch up on current news and reminisce, too. When our partners catch us belly-laughing at some old memory or private joke, they may want to be in on it. Because it's between the two of you, it may be inexplainable to others because "You just had to be there." These private jokes and childhood memories are precious; when you have the time to relive them with a good friend, do so!

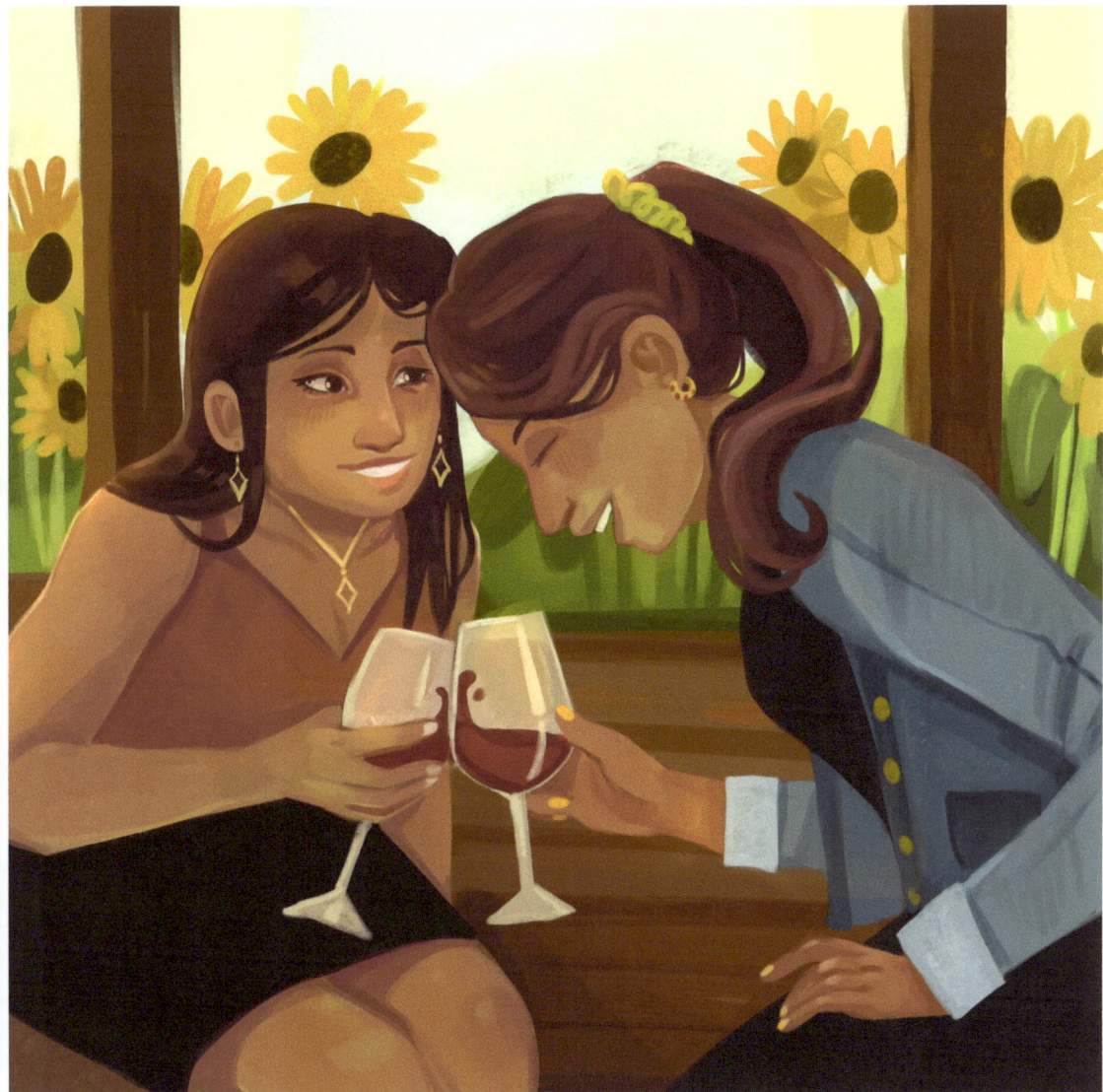

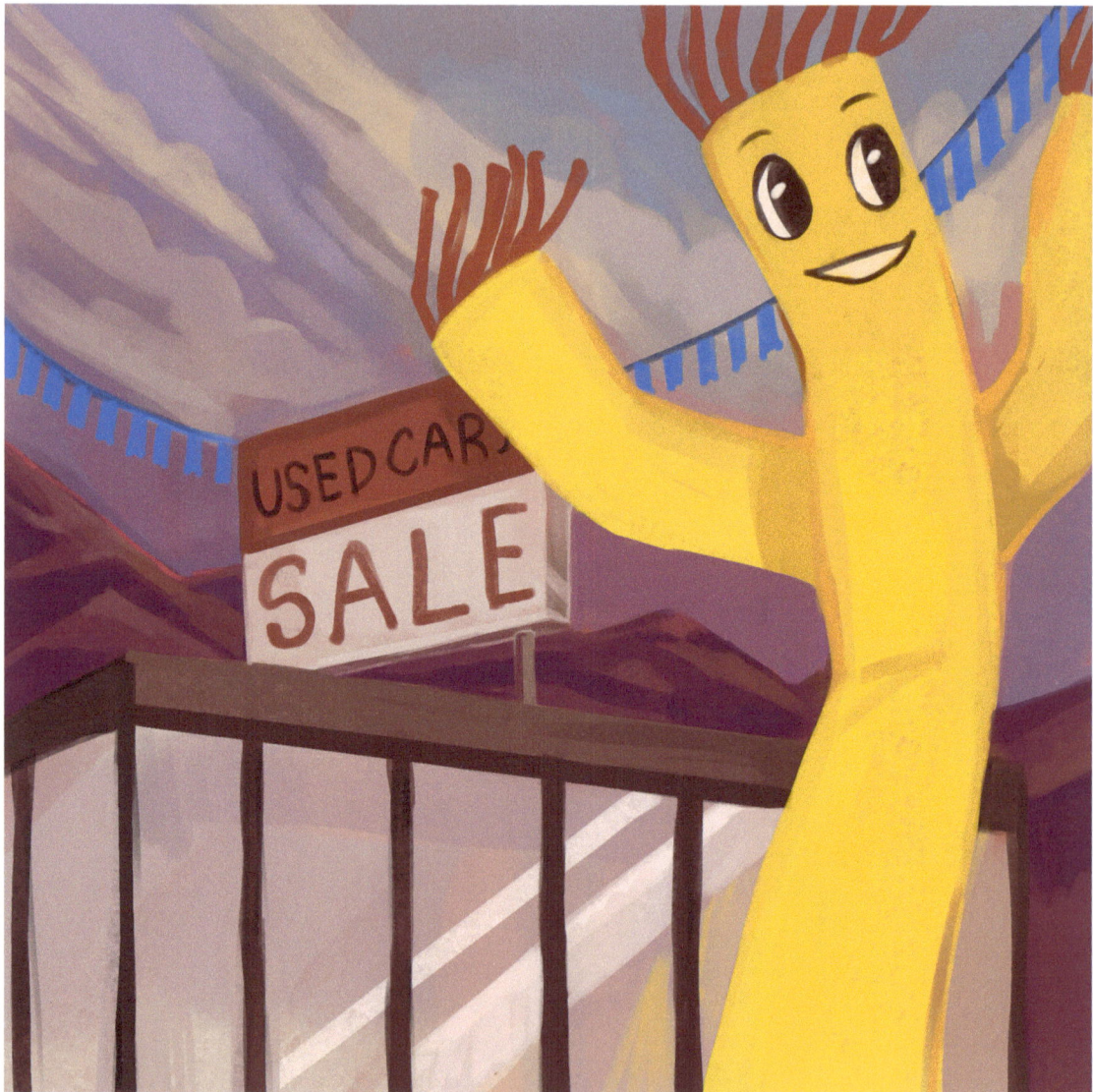

40

Act as junior mechanic or salesperson

If my husband is out of town and I'm bringing a car in to be serviced, I will consider asking a friend to go with me, especially if I don't know the dealership or shop. I feel like I have a sign on my head that says, "Sell me everything you offer, whether I need it or not." Our dad taught us the seven vital fluids of a car and basic car maintenance, but that is as far as I go. Bringing a knowledgeable friend with you when buying or servicing a car brings peace of mind to those times (and a relief for your wallet).

41

Offer pet care or plant care

A gardening friend loves to travel, and instead of worrying about the plants dying while she is gone, she will put some of her watering on timers, but more importantly trade care with another gardening friend. When she travels, she gives a key to that friend who knows how to take care of her indoor plants. When that friend travels, she takes care of her gardens. They don't exchange money. When friends are traveling, offer to take care of their pets, or plants, deliveries, or just checking on their home. It adds a little component of safety and care while they're gone.

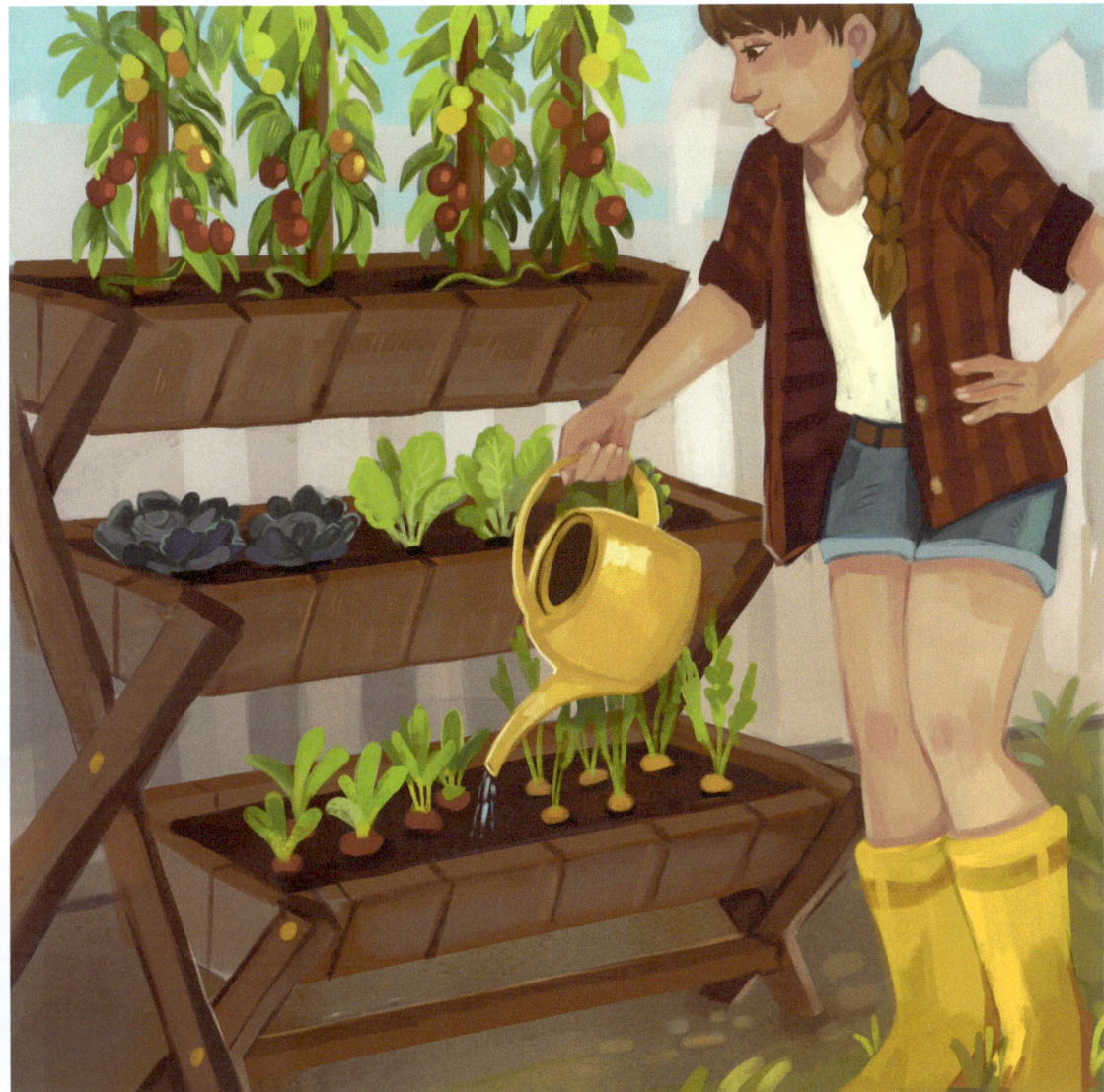

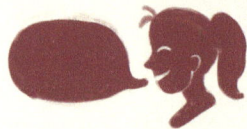

42

Share podcasts

When you're in your own head, the same ideas are recapitulated. You may have a deeper understanding of your perspective, but you likely need external information to make better decisions and act. Ask friends and colleagues who they trust for podcasters, news shows, play lists, YouTube® channels, and other sources of expertise. One of my favorite things to do is ask friends in other countries who they are following—I may never have found them without their recommendations, as many are not advertised in the US. These also offer a connection point when I'm traveling.

43

Buy or make "team friend" shirts

No one wants a medical malady to hit themselves or their
family, especially without an outside support system. When
you learn of a friend's personal challenge, offer to make or
buy "BFF" or "Team Friend" shirts to show you care. If she's
OK with the show of public support and announcing her issue
(a diagnosis, for example), gift them to everyone who is part
of the battle. Go with her to support groups. Take a picture
together. Join fundraisers for her or the cause in general.
With bright colors or goofy designs, you provide a welcome
distraction that may be surprisingly good for her spirits.

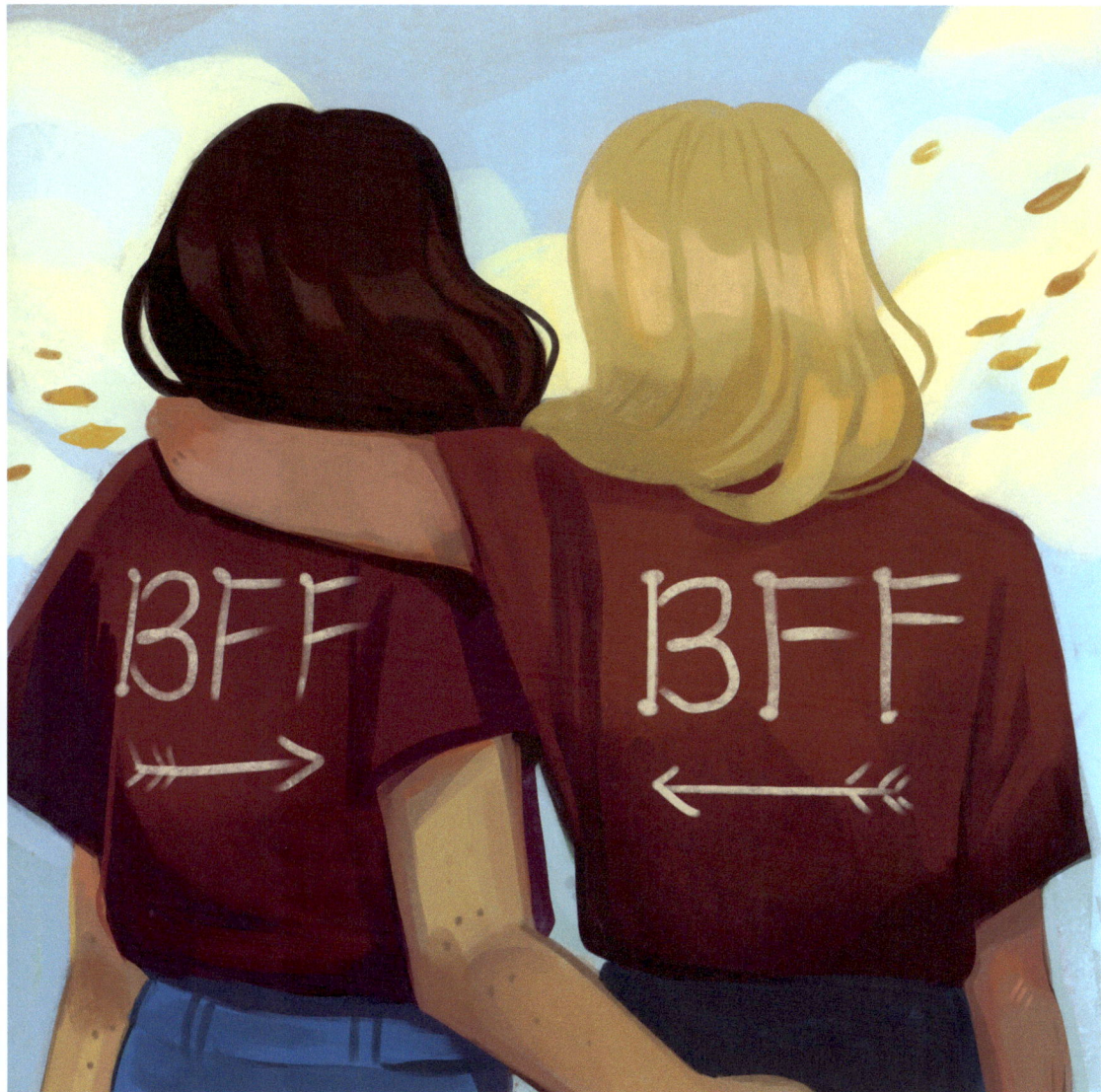

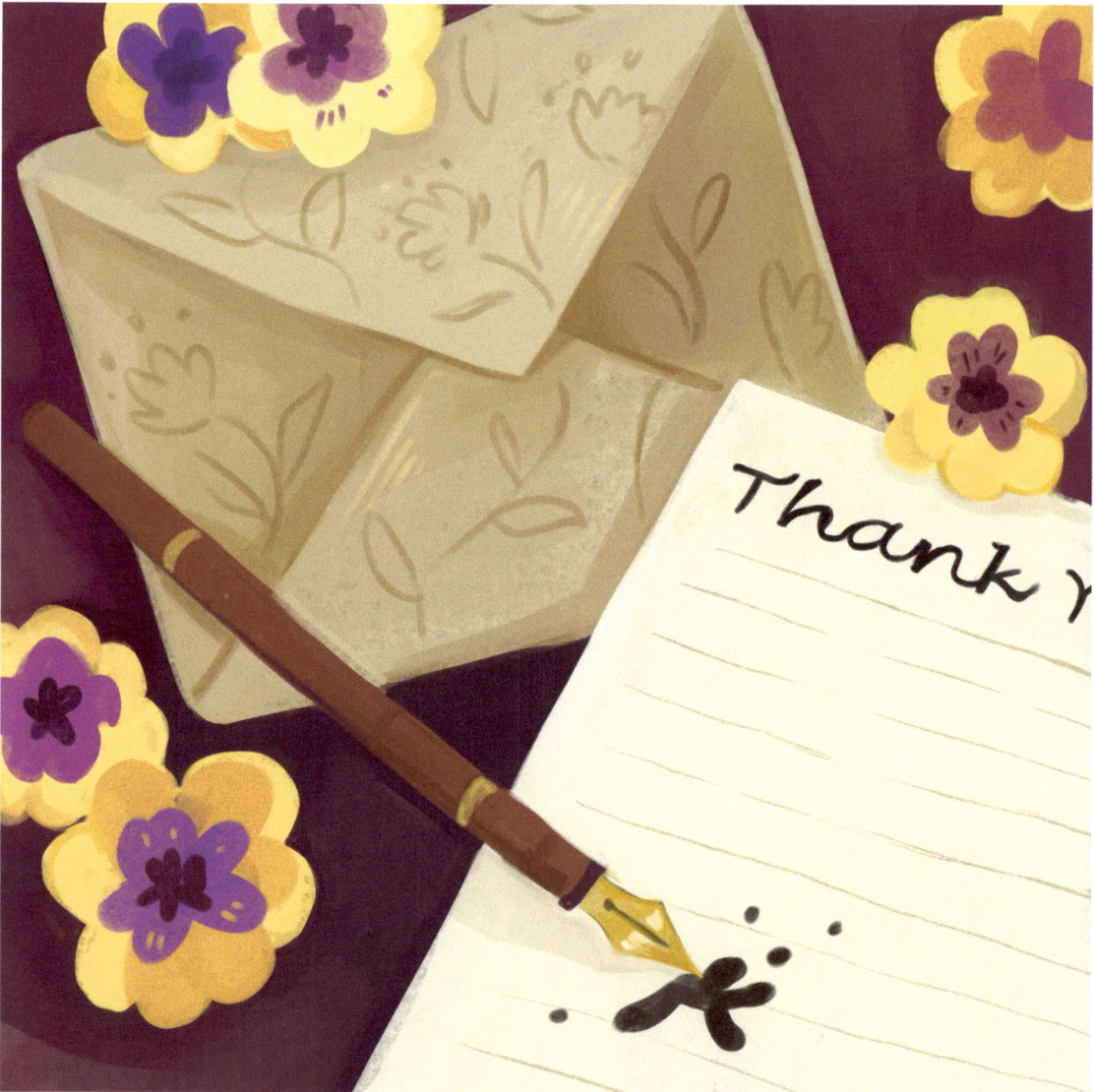

44

Hand-write notes

You can shoot them a quick text, send an email, or leave a voicemail, but nothing communicates quite like a handwritten card. While it takes a little longer and involves finding stationery and a stamp, it's worth it. After moving to a new city, I especially appreciated the thank you note from a new friend who followed up on our coffee chat. I kept that card on my desk for three months as an inspiration when I was going to head out to new events where I knew no one. You never know what inspiration your hand-written card will have.

45

Organize the garage or craft room

Recently, a young woman shared with me how she organized her craft room. She bought an adjustable rack mount for her yarn, then bought 16 inexpensive clear tub-like containers (same size) for her other craft supplies. With an equally-crafty friend, she divided them into categories. Then, they used a labeling machine to be more specific on contents, and stacked them alphabetically to make finding things more efficient. They had so much fun comparing stories about what they had made with the individual supplies, and then they decided to trade remnants with each other!

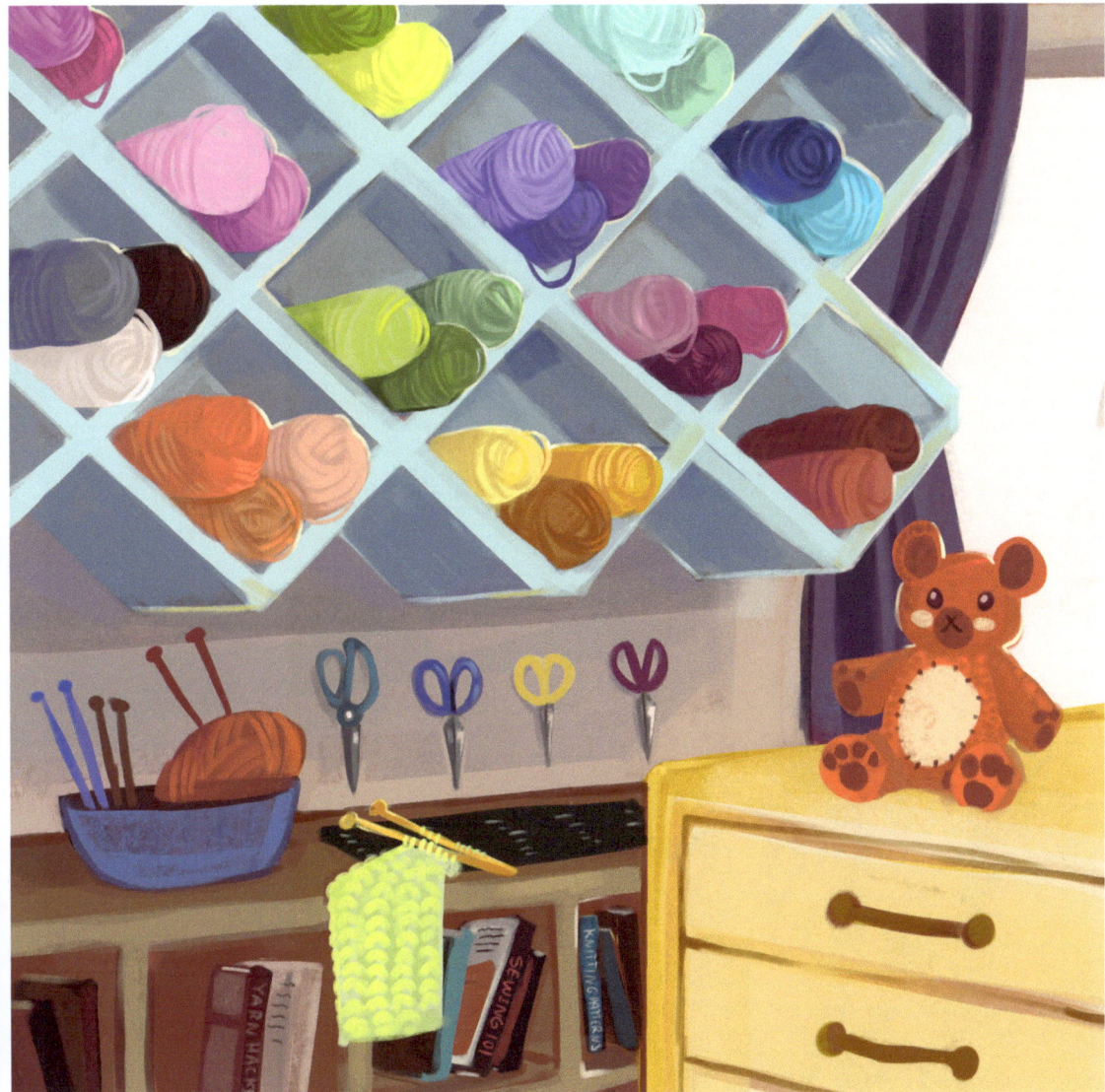

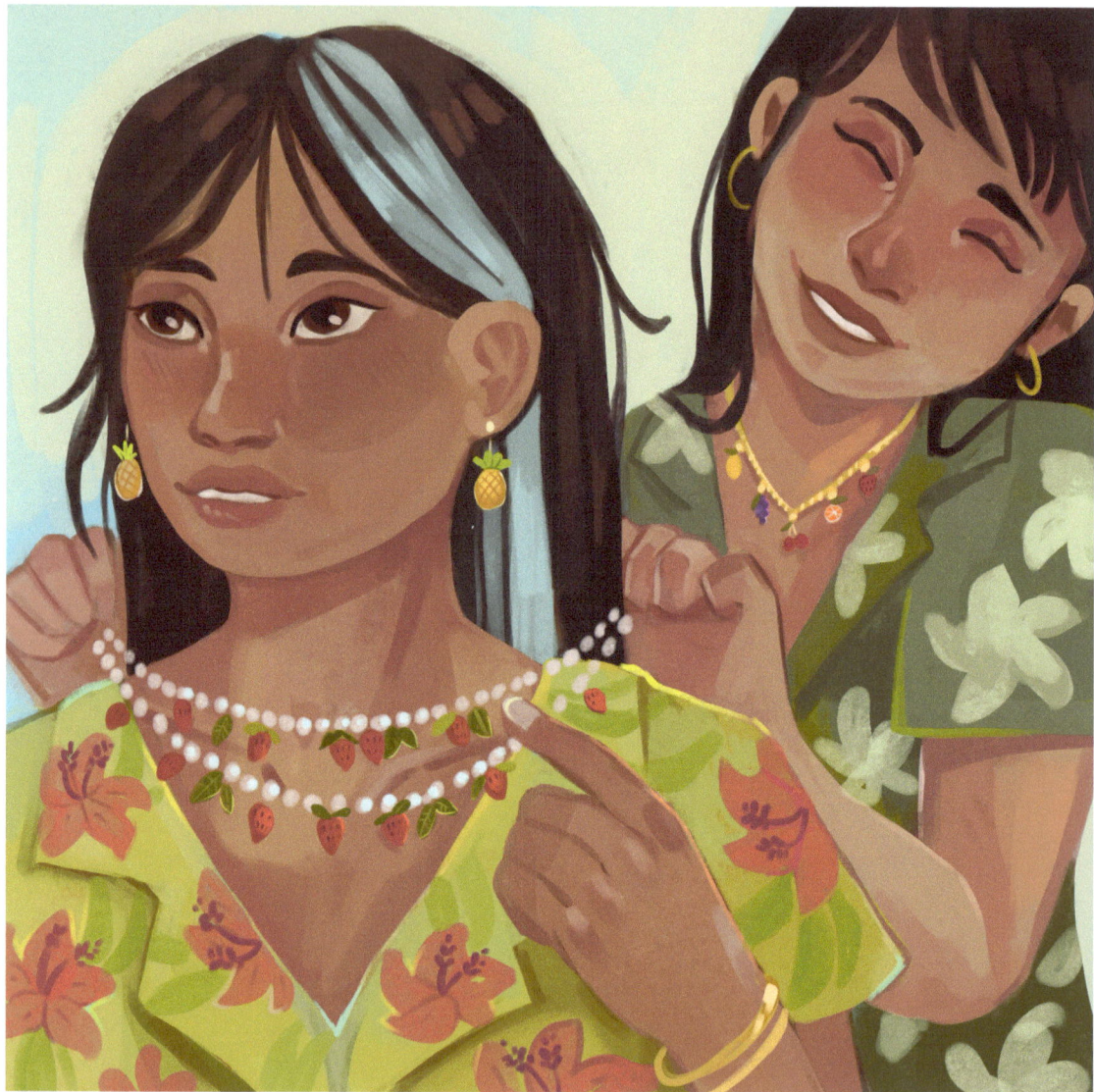

46

Borrow jewelry

You've always coveted your best friend's colorful necklace, perfect for many spring outfits. You've tried to find one for yourself to no avail. What about borrowing it? You could hint, ask to try it on, or say, "Saturday's my event and it would go great with my floral dress. Could I borrow it?" If it's not too expensive or has too much sentimental value, chances are she would let you borrow it. Remember to return it in as good or better shape than you got it by wiping it off and securing it in its box or bag. Be sure to share any compliments you receive!

47

Let them know you're thinking of them

Every time I see Brazilian coffee, food, or pastries, I think of a dear friend from Brazil. She introduced me to the wonderful world of Brazilian coffee, Brigadeiros pastries, and cheese bread. She even encouraged me to travel there! Since we no longer live in the same city, I can't share those with her in person, but I feel like she's with me when I buy them on my own, in a restaurant or Brazillian shop. I'll let her know I was thinking about her, I miss her, and I look forward to catching up.

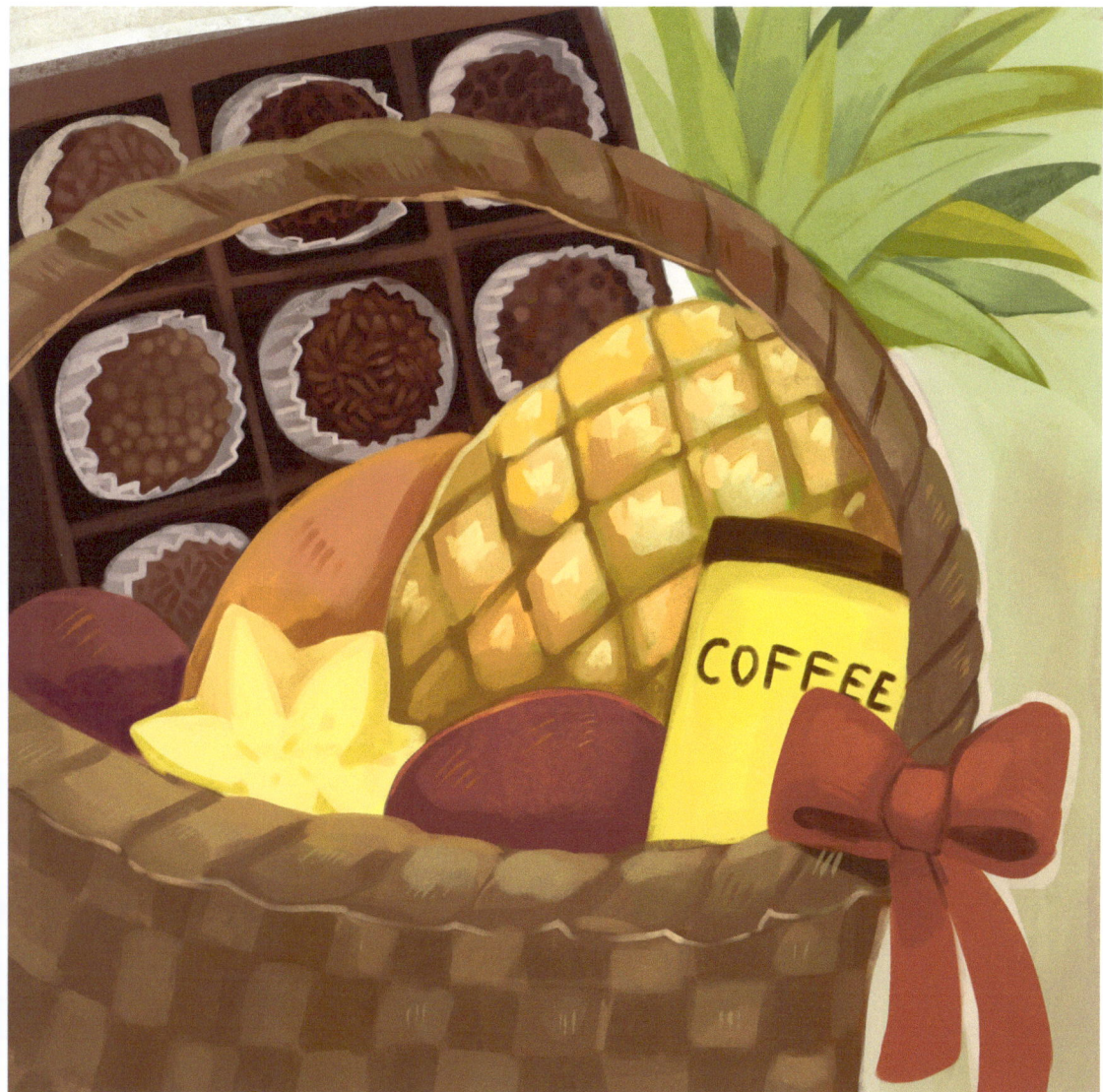

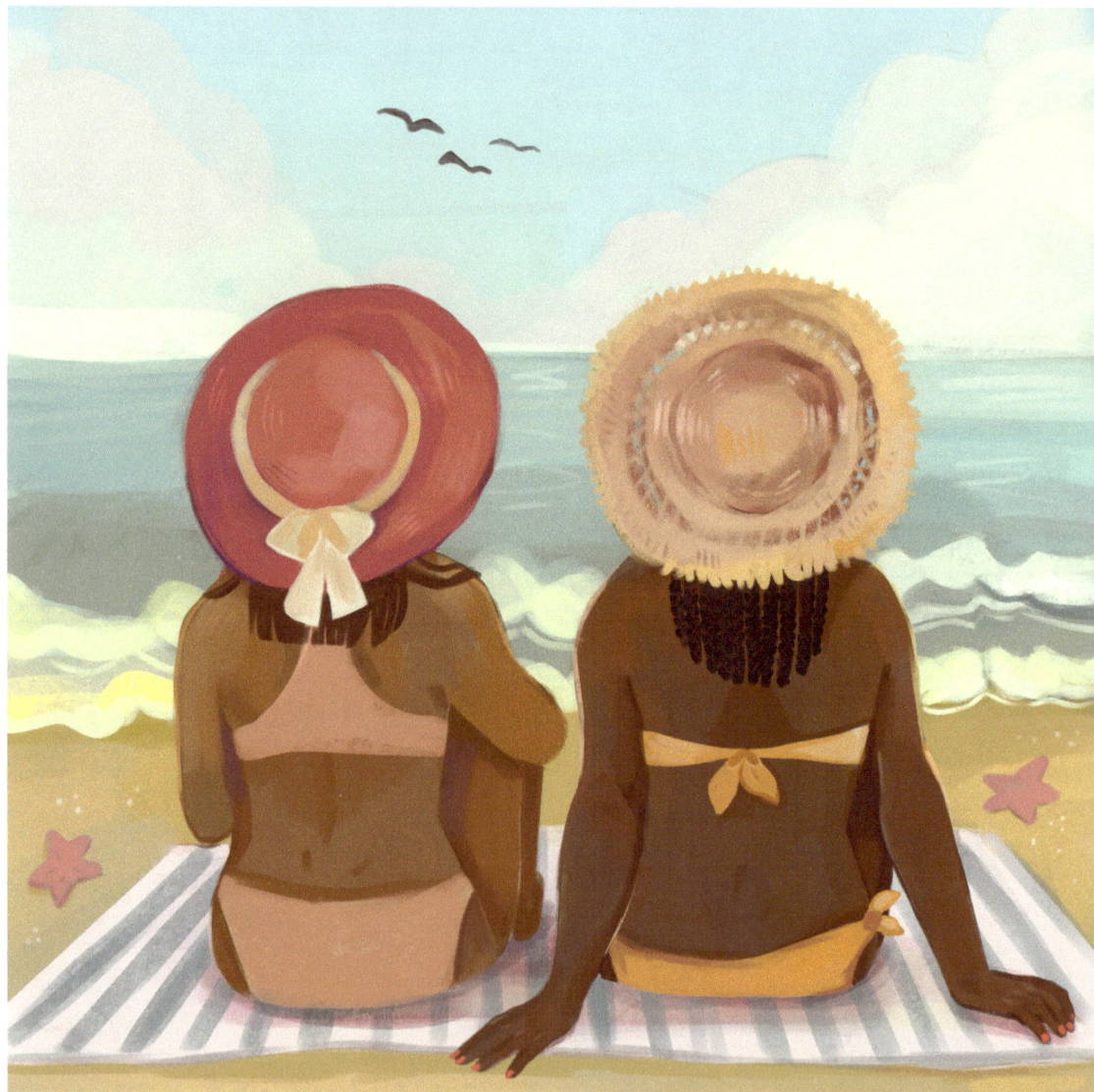

48

Time your tanning

When you're laying out by the pool, in your back yard or the beach, watch out for each other's skin. In college, we used to joke about setting our 15-minute timer, announcing, "It's time to turn so you don't burn!" Now it's more like, "Where's your hat and sunglasses to protect your face?" Friends will let you know when you've been out in the sun too long, and help with spraying sunscreen on hard-to-reach places. They also may recommend fun magazines or books to read while relaxing, especially those with sunny, summertime themes!

49

Enjoy the outdoors

Share the beauty and majesty of Mother Nature. Walk on a paved path or unpaved trail just for the sake of being with each other in the outdoors. Saunter by a waterfall, have a picnic, bird watch, rent a canoe, or see an arboretum exhibit. As I've often said, wordless walking, taking in the grandeur of your surroundings, is hard to surpass for relaxation and feeling close. Taking a break from being indoors and connected to technology feels good, and sharing it with someone who feels the same—without needing to have it explained—is priceless.

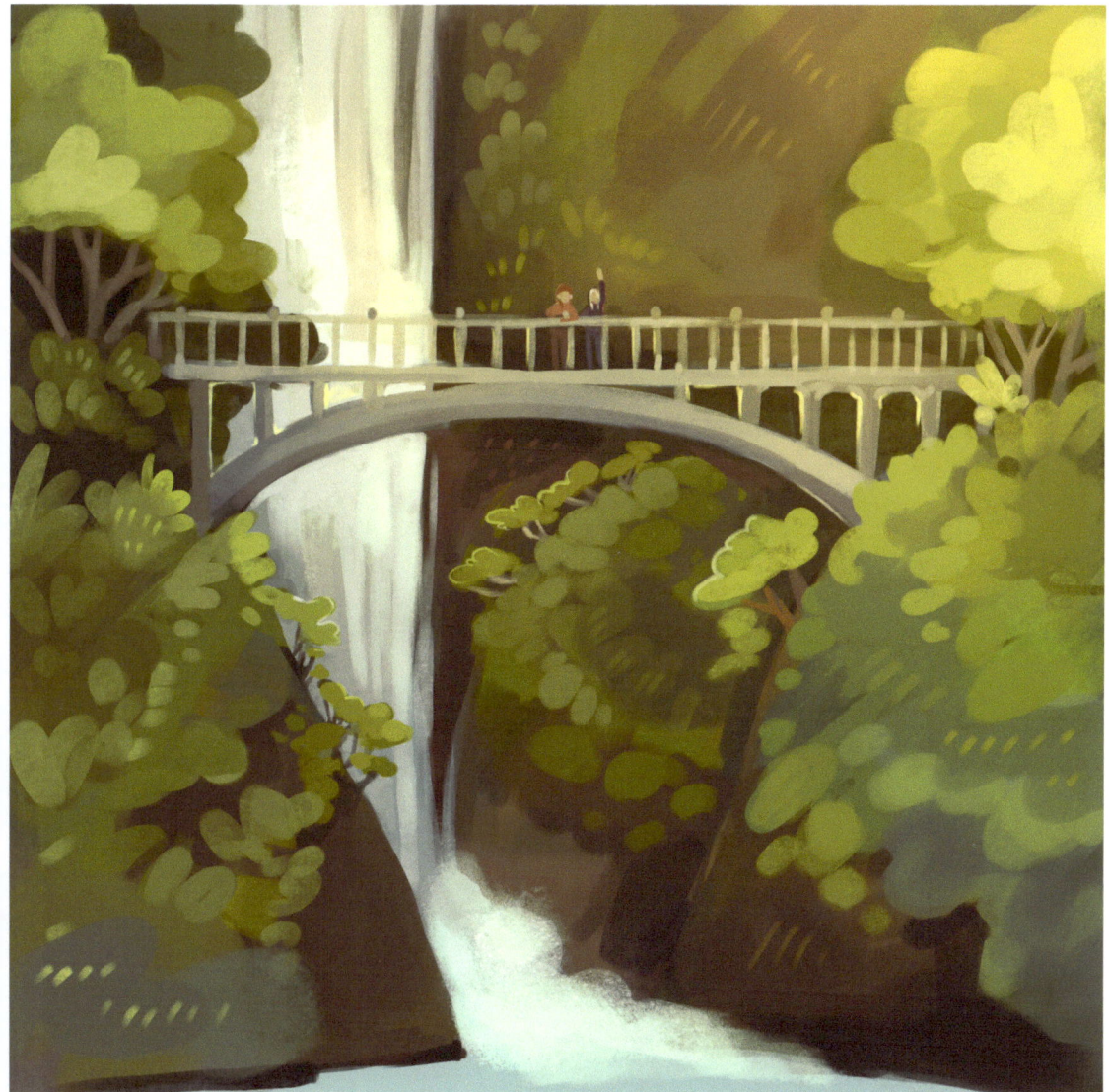

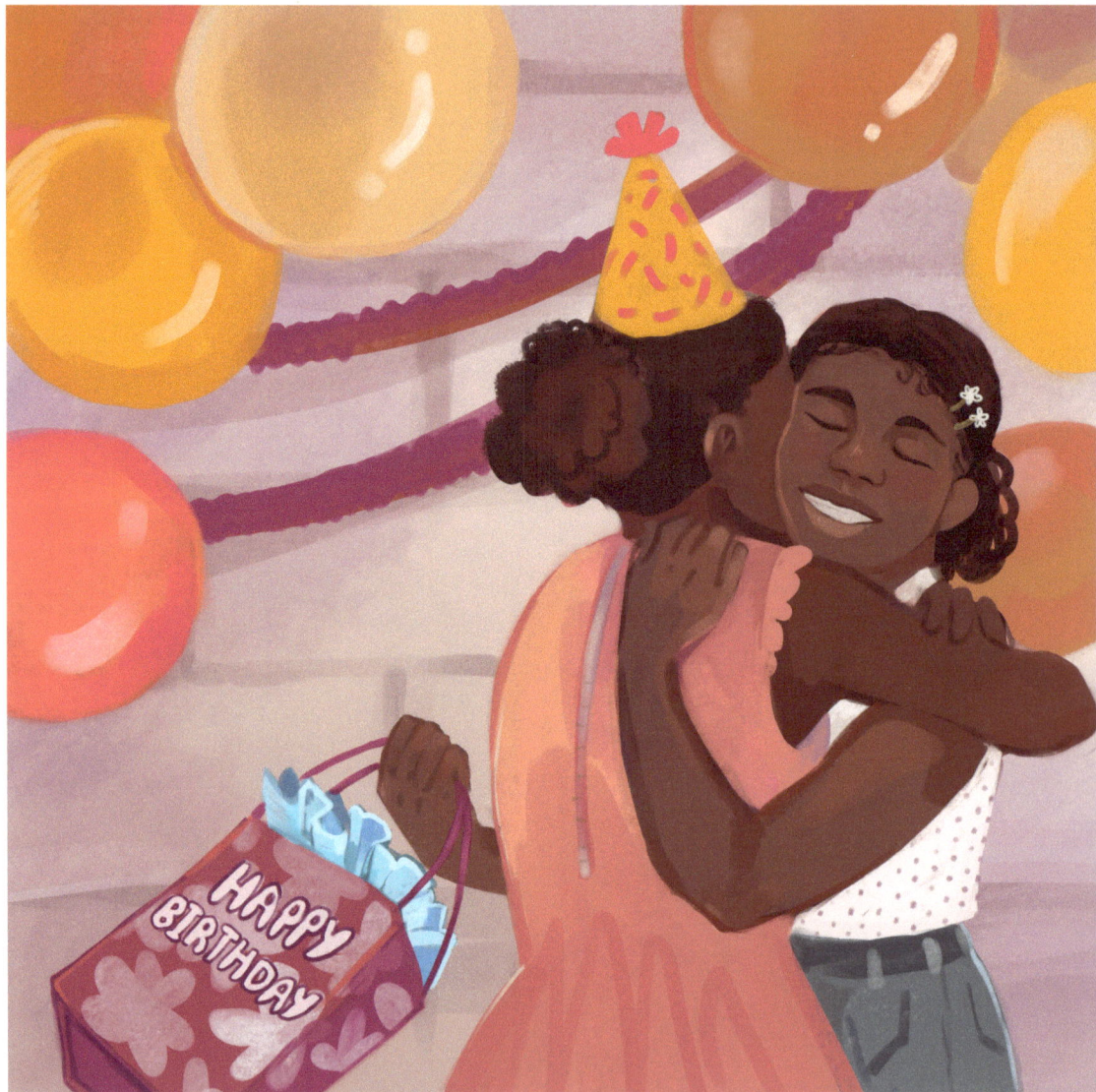

50

Celebrate or commiserate with a hug

When there are no words—for challenges or celebrations—a hug is the often the best solution. Being enveloped with nonjudgmental, caring arms is a blessing. Good friends have the innate understanding of when to be present. When the focus needs to be all about you. When to love on you and listen. It may be hard to articulate what you need from one situation to the next, happy or sad. Emotional responses are not a one-size-fits-all situation. Friends, especially close ones, seem to know this and give good hugs, maybe also asking later, "What do you need?"

51

Make massage appointments

If you have just helped someone move, clean out a closet, organize the garage, or bake a bunch of cookies (or other suggestions in this book), you may feel a bit achy and sore—and so may she. That's the perfect time to suggest a massage. With so many options available such as short head-shoulders-neck version to two hours deep tissue, you may be able to schedule one that fits into your time and budget. After you've done something satisfying together and then gotten a good massage, it's hard to not feel terrific. It's also a nice way to say "thank you" to them for helping you out.

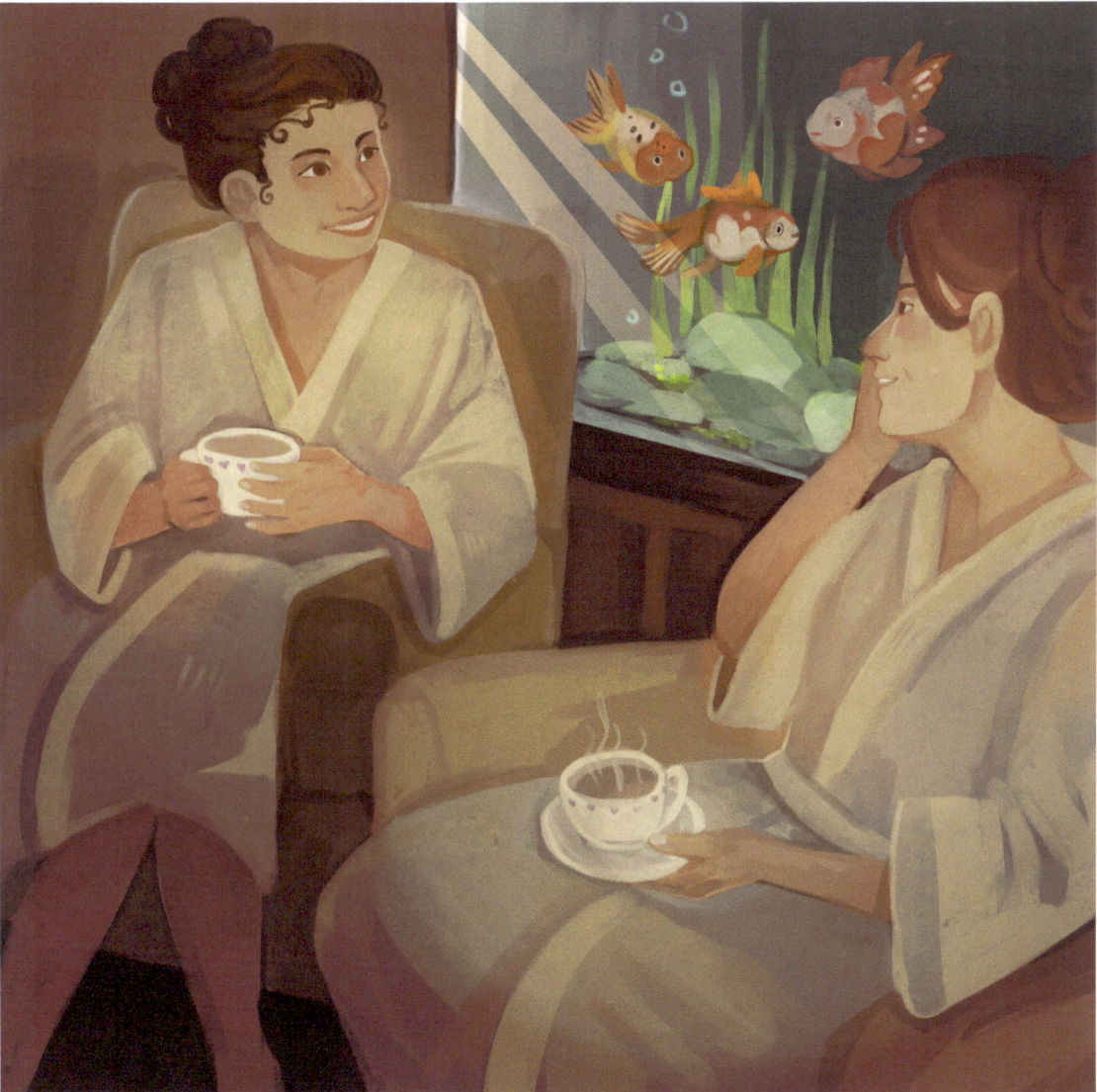

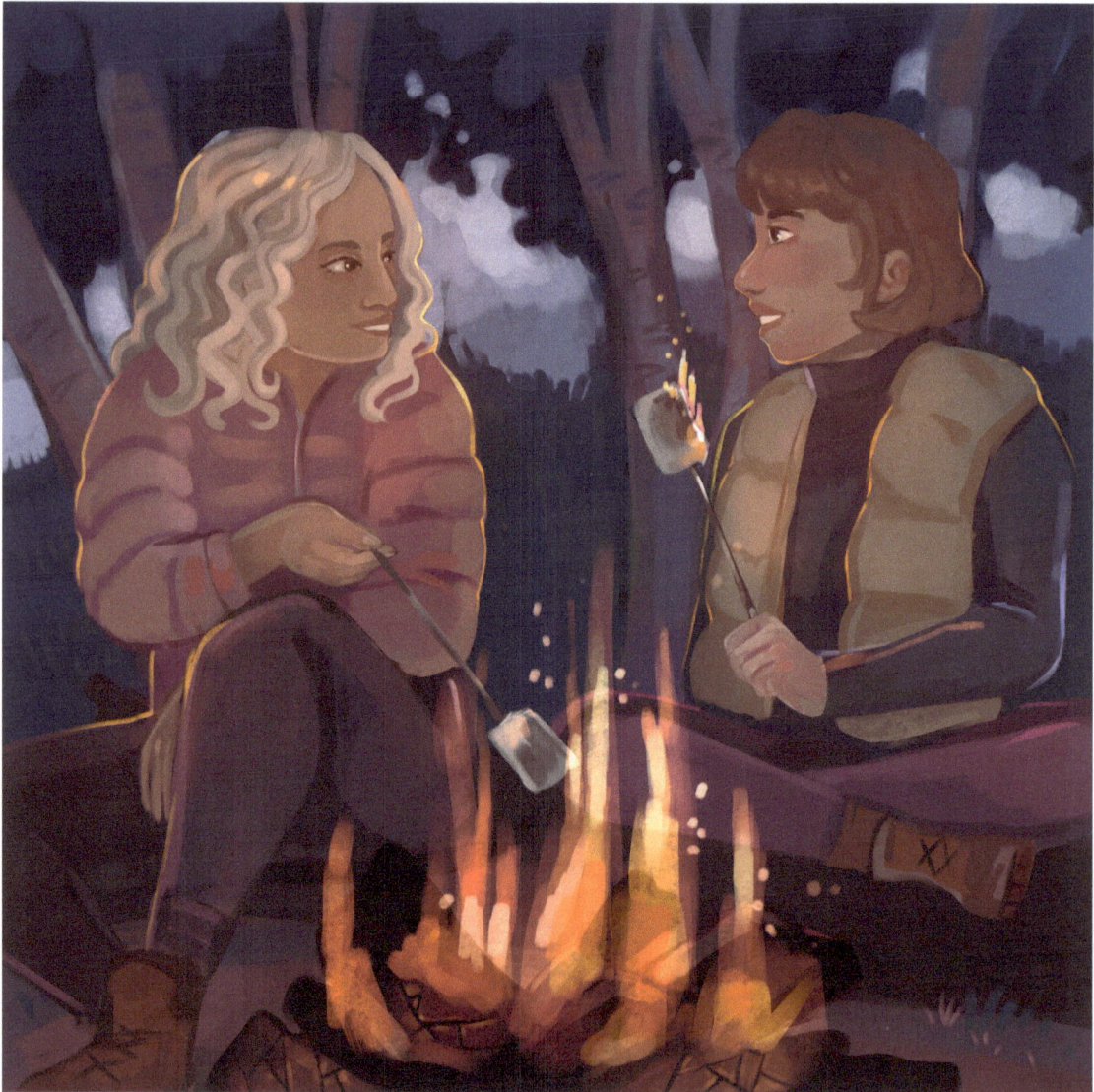

52

Say, "You're a great friend. Thank you."

November is extra special for me, as I use part of every day to thank those who have shown up for me during the year. It's a practice you could consider: write an email to your special people (it may be a little hard to find 30 of them) to tell them you're thankful and why. Let them know they matter to you, and what they do is meaningful and appreciated. When you thank a wonderful friend or business colleague for being on this journey of life with you, the side benefit is strengthening that relationship. It may be the nicest message they get all year!

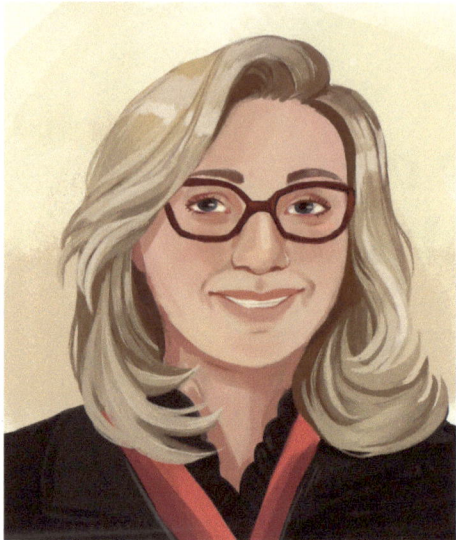

About the Author

A lifelong learner and writer, Bonnie B. Daneker has been part of the publishing industry for more than 20 years. She established Georgia's first publishing advisory firm to help clients write books and has managed over 100 book-content projects.

Before her time in publishing, she worked in technology consulting. Bonnie holds a BA in Journalism from The Ohio State University, an MBA in Strategic Planning and Entrepreneurship from The Goizueta Business School at Emory University, and the Sustainability Associate Certification from ISSP. She has instructed at Savannah College of Art and Design (SCAD) and guest-lectured at Emory University. Bonnie lives with her husband outside Dallas, TX.

Visit her website at www.TheAuthorsGreenhouse.com

About the Illustrator

A "digital painter," Eevie Lanier is a book and visual development illustrator. She has done work for Square Panda and Stride educational video games.

Eevie is a graduate of Savannah College of Art and Design(SCAD) with a BFA in Illustration with a Concentration in Concept Design for Animation and Games. Previously, she graduated from the Alabama School of Fine Arts. She lives in Birmingham, AL with her two dogs and one cat.

She can be reached through LinkedIn at: www.linkedin.com/in/Eevie-Lanier.

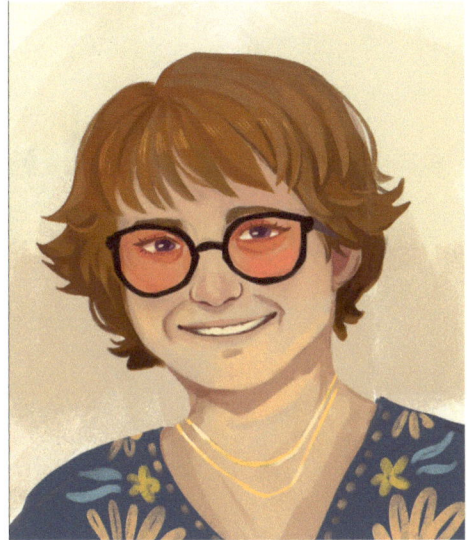

More from
Bonnie B. Daneker:

———————————

Stoplights Are For Kissing

Stoplights Are For Singing

Leave a Review!

———————————

As a self-published author, reviews mean the world! Please leave a review on the platform from which you purchased this book. I read every one!

www.ingramcontent.com/pod-product-compliance
Lightning Source LLC
Chambersburg PA
CBHW041240020426
42333CB00002B/23

* 9 7 8 0 9 9 1 0 0 3 2 5 9 *